A SYSTEMS APPROACH TO ALCOHOL TREATMENT

ERRATA: see pp. 304 - 305.

A SYSTEMS APPROACH TO ALCOHOL TREATMENT

by

FREDERICK B. GLASER, M.D.

STEPHANIE W. GREENBERG, M.A.

and

MORRIS BARRETT, M.P.H.

With Forewords By

James G. Rankin, M.D. and Robert E. Popham
Addiction Research Foundation

and

Morris E. Chafetz, M.D., Former Director
National Institute on Alcohol Abuse and Alcoholism

ADDICTION RESEARCH FOUNDATION
Toronto, Canada

Permission to publish this book has been granted by the Governor's Council on Drug and Alcohol Abuse of the Commonwealth of Pennsylvania, which supported this work under contract. However, the opinions expressed are those of the authors and do not necessarily reflect the opinions of the Governor's Council.

ISBN: 0-88868-025-2

Printed in Canada.

This book is dedicated to

ARTHUR DONALD MOFFETT

1941 - 1974

What I must do is die now. I must accept
the justice of death and the injustice of life.
I have lived a good life —
longer than many, better than most. . . .
I have had
thirty-three years. I couldn't ask for another
day. What did I do to deserve birth?
It was a gift. I am me—that is a miracle.
I had no right to a single minute. Some
are given a single hour. And yet I have had
thirty-three years.

—Hugh Prather

Table of Contents

Foreword

by
Morris E. Chafetz, M.D.
Former Director
National Institute on Alcohol Abuse and Alcoholism

Public ambivalence, misconception, and moral biases toward alcohol use and alcoholism have greatly influenced the manner in which alcoholism treatment facilities have developed in this country. A tragic myth that alcoholic people cannot be and do not want to be treated is still operating in the minds of many people, even some of the people who are responsible for delivering treatment and care for alcoholic individuals. The often unaccepted truth is that alcoholic people respond very well to quality treatment. We can treat alcoholism at least as successfully as most other illnesses which are common.

The authors of this volume have addressed an urgent situation—the fact that existing treatment facilities are not servicing the vast majority of the alcoholic population. This comprehensive, State-wide evaluation of alcoholism treatment centers has also indicated that a coordinated treatment service system did not exist within the State of Pennsylvania. Let me point out, however, that this is not a unique situation in perspective of the status of such systems either in other States or in the Nation as a whole.

Generally, the failure of such treatment systems has been due to a variety of factors, the most obvious being that primary focus is too often on the public inebriate or skidrow alcoholic, a person who only represents five percent of those in need of help for alcohol problems. Other reasons for failure have been because of a restricted outlook in approach to treatment and an emphasis on only one type of service such as maintenance. Limited knowledge of the resources, programs, and procedures of other available health agencies, institutionalized inefficiency, and a general insensitivity to the physical and psychological needs of alcoholic people have also limited program success. A most disturbing factor is that many programs have failed because all too often, they have consumed limited resources by responding largely to themselves, instead of to the needs of desperately ill people.

I feel that this book exhibits a challenge to all of us in the field of alcoholism in that it asks us to re-examine our primary commitment to helping alcoholic people. More specifically, it presented to the Governor's Council on Drug and Alcohol Abuse a factual base from which to proceed toward developing a systematic alcoholism service delivery program in the State of Pennsylvania.

Foreword

by

James G. Rankin
Director, Clinical Institute

Robert E. Popham
Director, Research Division

Addiction Research Foundation of Ontario

There is growing concern in North America and other industrialized societies about the increasing size, complexity, and cost of health services; and it is clear that there is an increasing demand that whatever services are provided in future relate to a demonstrated need and are both effective and efficient in meeting the need.

The expansion of services for the treatment and rehabilitation of persons with problems attributable to excessive alcohol use has been particularly noticeable since the early 1960s. While this is not the first time that there has been an increased effort to provide health care for such persons, generally speaking, as in the past, the effort has been unsystematic and to date has not had an appreciable impact on the evolution of an economical and effective response to the problem. Clearly a new approach is required which will assure that all elements of health care delivery are systematically tested, and altered in accord with the results to the end that a fully rational utilization of resources ultimately may be achieved.

A Systems Approach to Alcohol Treatment demonstrates the general condition of the relevant resources in Pennsylvania circa 1973. But the situation in that state obtains throughout North America and probably in other industrialized nations as well. The picture presented is anything but reassuring.

Over the past 20 years, there have been positive developments in the field of alcohol problems. There has been a general acceptance of alcoholism as a health problem; an increase in knowledge with regard to the nature, prevention, and management of alcohol problems; and an increased demand for the provision of treatment resources with a more or less commensurate response to this demand by government and private groups.

Nevertheless, the response which evolved in Pennsylvania was fragmentary and uncoordinated, and there was absolutely no scientifically valid knowledge as to how effective the various programs were. The results of the study in these respects are similar to those reported for such other North American areas as Alaska, North Carolina, the State of Washington, and Ontario, Canada. The study showed that services were available at any point in time to only approximately 1% of the population in need. What was being provided appeared to have no relationship to measures of need or knowledge of treatment techniques, and there was little evidence of cooperation among the many individual programs. The level of the response in a particular area appeared to be influenced mainly by factors other than need — for example, chance occurences, opportunity, and interest. The approach to treatment was entrepreneurial in character and tended to reflect the background or bias of the staff. Treatment programs rather than being comprehensive were extremely limited.

In describing the situation with regard to problems of alcohol use, attention should also be drawn to a previously published companion study which demonstrated that the situation with regard to the treatment of individuals with drug problems had been essentially the same.*

Although there is every reason for major concern about the present state of resources for the care of alcohol or drug damaged individuals, it is important to avoid the mistake of believing that this is the only area for which health care is not based on sound knowledge, logic, and planning. In many other areas of health care there are problems resulting from the separateness rather than the interdependence of treatment resources — from the failure to tailor the treatment approach to the individual needs of patients, from the disparity between scientific knowledge and treatment, and in general, from the lack of a sequential approach to health problems based on effective detection, assessment, and referral for specifically tailored interventions. Problems of this nature can be identified even in the response to relatively less complex health concerns such as breast cancer and hypertension, but become much more pronounced when the attempt is made to cope with such concerns as mental retardation, mental disorders, alcoholism, and drug dependence.

The authors conclude their study by proposing a "core-shell" treatment system which is eminently worthy of careful examination as a way to overcome the principal deficiencies in current treatment approaches to the problems of alcohol use. In fact, under the direction of the senior author, Dr. Frederick Glaser, this system has recently been implemented at the Clinical Institute of the Addiction Research Foundation in Toronto, where it is being intensively studied. It is evident that the concepts embodied in the system are applicable to the management of other drug-related problems as well, and quite probably to health care delivery in general, as a potential means to assure the rational evolution of an increasingly effective and efficient system.

* *A Systems Approach to Drug Treatment* by Fred Adler, Arthur D. Moffett, Frederick B. Glaser, John C. Ball, and Diana Horvitz. Philadelphia: Dorrance 1974, xvi & 328 pp.

Finally, it should be stressed that the authors have not considered the question of treatment in isolation from other approaches to resolving problems of alcohol use. Thus, they give attention also to the role of public and professional education, and to government policy in relation to the prevention of alcoholism. In the latter connection, much of the argument is based on the studies of the effects of legal control measures conducted by the Addiction Research Foundation of Ontario.

We would like to commend the authors for a very superior piece of research, indeed a model of the type of examination of health services which should be carried out in other jurisdictions. The authors were about as rigorous in their survey as could be reasonably expected in so complex an area. They are highly objective in reporting their results and have exercised commendable restraint in drawing conclusions. Perhaps most importantly, they have not merely made a diagnosis, but have proposed what is proving to be a useful and productive remedy.

Acknowledgments

A large number of organizations and individuals provided the authors with essential assistance throughout the work on this project. Our thanks most of all must go to the directors and staff members of the alcoholism treatment programs of the Commonwealth of Pennsylvania. They gave unstintingly of their time and freely of their knowledge, and made our little band feel welcome and at home throughout the thousands of arduous miles we necessarily had to travel. We hope that our work will be of help to them. Our thanks extend also to the executive directors and MH/MR specialists in each county or joinder who assisted us in our task.

Many members of the staff of the Section on Drug and Alcohol Abuse provided essential support to the project. Most of all, and although he cannot now know it, we should like to thank the late Arthur Moffett, who participated in virtually all of the site visits. Art was in many ways the very soul of the project, and indeed of all that we did. He is sadly missed. Freda Adler, Diana Horvitz, and DiAnne Walters also participated in the field work. Mary Connelly, Wanda Boyd, and Helen Constantine provided invaluable secretarial assistance in preparing the many drafts of the manuscript. Deena Watson and May McReynolds assumed many additional responsibilities so this work might be completed and helped immeasureably in the final assembly of the manuscript.

At Eastern Pennsylvania Psychiatric Institute, where the SDAA lived and worked, Ulysses Watson, Bernard Borislow, and William Wescott provided both administrative and moral support. Ruby Horwood, librarian of the Institute, and her staff provided invaluable bibliographic assistance and were most patient with the many demands which the project engendered. At the Medical College of Pennsylvania, of whose department of psychiatry the SDAA was a part, Leo Madow, Lawrence Snow, and Robert Slater were a constant source of encouragement.

Richard Horman of the Governor's Council on Drug and Alcohol Abuse was administratively responsible for this study. The members and consultants of the Governor's Council are to be thanked for their support of the project. Other staff of the Governor's Council, including Peter Pennington, George Taylor, Thomas Keil, Frances Baker Dickman, Holly Gardner, and Lou Grimaldi especially were extremely helpful in many ways. Our thanks also go to many members of the staff of the regional offices of the Council.

Although our knowledge of Philadelphia, the home base of the SDAA, allowed us to navigate there with little more than the general support of John Riggan and his excellent staff, their cheerful and pleasant helpfulness was appreciated. In Pittsburgh, with its great array of programs, we would have been lost without assistance. We would particularly like to thank Gloria Stubbs for all her efforts on our behalf. George Lowe, Stephen Lenhart, and Annette Green also helped us greatly.

Morris E. Chafetz and John Deering formerly of the National Institute on Alcohol Abuse and Alcoholism were most helpful, and Dr. Chafetz also provided a Foreword. The Robert Wood Johnson Foundation and the Institute of Medicine are to be thanked for permitting one of the authors to take time out from a fellowship year in Washington to work on the final manuscript. The staffs of the Library of the College of Physicians of Philadelphia and of the Library Company of Philadelphia were of particular assistance in preparing the historical portion of the manuscript. Robert Popham of the Addiction Research Foundation in Toronto provided invaluable advice and assistance in the preparation of the report on the state liquor monopoly, and he and Dr. James G. Rankin of the Foundation's Clinical Institute also provided a Foreword. Barbara Rutledge, managing editor of the Foundation, performed an invaluable service by editing a long and complex manuscript.

Finally and most importantly, the authors would like to thank their husbands, wives, and children for their understanding of the importance of this work and for their forbearance in the face of the many hours devoted to it. Their faith, as exemplified by this investment, augured well for the ultimate success of the project.

The Authors
July, 1977

Introduction
To This Book and Its Uses

The best way to avoid confusion in thinking about the ways of human beings is to remember that the number of ideas that have really moved mankind is very small and most of this small number of ideas is very simple. The difficulty is that you and I have room in our heads for only one or two of these simple ideas at the same time.

—*The Ramayana*

As lengthy as it is, and as filled with figures, charts, tables, and appendices as it may be, this book really tells a rather simple tale. A group of interested people wanted to find out what was being done in terms of the treatment of alcoholism in Pennsylvania. Therefore they visited all of the programs which were performing this service. They saw much that was good. But they found that there was no overall coherence and unified thrust to the effort. It was fragmented, entrepreneurial, redundant, and discontinuous; in short, there was no treatment system.

That, in essence, is the whole tale; and one who wishes only a general knowledge of the thesis of the work may stop reading at once. All else that is here simply fills in this general picture in greater detail. The large amount of detail is provided so that those who wish to do so may make an independent judgment as to whether the data gathered in fact support the conclusions which have been drawn. To facilitate this process, the book has been divided into four sections. The sections bear a logical and sequential relationship to each other, but they have been written so that they may be read independently with maximum comprehension. This is also true of the individual chapters which comprise the four sections.

Section One of the book contains both general and specific introductory material. The first chapter provides a broad historical perspective on the use and abuse of alcohol in Pennsylvania and the manner in which it was dealt with prior to the period under study. In a sense, the chapter provides the overall context within which the specific study to be reported was carried out; but the study is capable of being understood on its own terms, and the eager reader may progress immediately to the study proper. This begins in the second chapter of Section One, in which the methodology of the study is explained.

Section Two presents both the data which were gathered in the course of the survey of treatment programs and the specific conclusions which were drawn from those data regarding the several aspects of treatment which were studied: the way the program directors thought about alcoholism itself; the goals which they set for their programs in dealing with it; the number and kinds of patients and staff in the programs; the facilities in which they were housed; their relationships to the community; the overall quality of the programs; and so forth. An attempt has been made to present primarily summary tables of the data in these chapters, with the more detailed data being relegated to an appendix. In addition, ample use has been made of charts and graphs to convey the essence of the findings.

Section Three includes some of the most interesting material which the authors encountered during the course of the survey. While the focus of the study was upon treatment programs, it soon became apparent that there were specific aspects of the general environment of the Commonwealth which had to be understood as well. A principal example of this is that extraordinary organization, Alcoholics Anonymous. No one could have an adequate grasp of the past, present, and future of alcoholism treatment in Pennsylvania without considerable knowledge of AA. Yet it was not possible for the research team, given its limited time frame and resources, to survey AA in the depth in which it surveyed the treatment programs. As a compromise, the team visited a small number of representative AA programs and studied the copious extant literature. The second chapter of Section Three is the result. All of the other chapters in the section were produced in a similar manner. Unlike the material in Section Two, the chapters here are *not* based upon a 100% sample but upon a much smaller and more selective sample, and are heavily buttressed by other data from the literature and from personal experience. Given this, the conclusions drawn in Section Three should perhaps be considered as rather more speculative than those to be found in Section Two. Future, more intensive studies of each of these areas may well be required.

Section Four presents a summary of the overall findings of the entire study, and the recommendations for future action which the authors view as flowing from these findings. Chapter 16, the summary chapter, includes a summary of Chapter 17, the recommendations chapter; thus those interested in a very rapid glimpse of the entire work may obtain this by reading Chapter 16 alone. A word of caution regarding conclusions and recommendations in general is in order. If the research team had followed the most rigorous scientific approach, only the data would have been presented and no conclusions would have been drawn; no recommendations would have been made. Basic science demands virtually no attempt to transcend the data. However, the authors have viewed this study as an exercise in applied science, specifically intended to be useful in the formulation of governmental policy. They have therefore gone ahead and drawn conclusions and made recommendations, while fully conscious of the many pitfalls involved in that speculative process. They feel that the data have been presented in sufficient detail to permit the interested reader to test whatever alternative conclusions may occur to him or her.

A large part of this detailed data may be found in the appendices. In addition, a directory of the treatment programs visited during the course of the survey has been included. This more precisely specifies the population of programs upon which the survey was based and provides a more detailed picture of individual treatment programs; all of the data contained in the chapters are aggregate in nature. Two pieces of basic legislation in the field of alcoholism are included as well. This is pursuant to a general impression of the survey team of a lack of familiarity of program personnel and others with these very basic documents which set limitations upon all that they do. Finally, both out of general interest and a desire for completeness on the one hand, and a wish to show how inextricably the problem of alcoholism is bound up with the operations of the government on the other hand, there is included a special report on the sale of alcohol through the state store system in Pennsylvania. This report was written during the time that a major study was being prepared for publication and hence is contemporaneous with it. In terms of approach it is even more heavily dependent upon scholarly research than the chapters of Section Three, though several state stores were visited during its course.

In sum, the book provides a reasonably comprehensive view of the overall effort of the Commonwealth of Pennsylvania in the field of alcoholism treatment at one point in its history, as seen through the eyes of an independent interdisciplinary research team which visited all of the relevant sites. There are many ways in which the interested reader may avail himself of these data. If he wishes to take the long approach, he will initially read another book by the same research group (*A Systems Approach to Drug Treatment,* by Freda Adler, Arthur D. Moffett, Frederick B. Glaser, John C. Ball, and Diana Horvitz, Philadelphia, Dorrance & Company, 1974). This book presents in considerably greater detail the development of the basic methodology of the present study, as well as its application to a cognate treatment system. He will then read the entire text and appendices of the current volume, together with those of the individual references which he may find to be critical.

On the other hand, if the press of business precludes such a thorough-going approach, a reader may look at as little as the first paragraph of this introduction or, if he has slightly more time, at Chapter 16 alone. There are also many intermediate pathways between these two extremes. One who reads Chapter 2 on the methodology of the study, Chapters 16 and 17 on the findings and recommendations, and whichever of the intervening chapters particularly interest him, will obtain an appreciable grasp of the substance of this volume. Of course it is hoped that many will have the time and/or inclination to peruse the entire volume.

Several caveats must be posted for the reader before he makes his selection of an approach to this material. First, he should recognize that this study does *not* provide a view of the Pennsylvania treatment system at the present time. The survey work was done during the calendar year 1973, and much has changed since then. In particular, the survey fails to reflect the impact which the single state agency charged with overall responsibility for alcoholism treatment (the Governor's Council on Drug and Alcohol Abuse) may have had. The Council was formed in mid-1972, and hence any major effect would not have been manifest while the field work was being done. In many ways this is extremely fortunate, for the book *does* provide a view of what the treatment system was like at the last possible moment prior to the impact of this agency. Hence it provides a baseline against which the effect of the agency may be judged at some future time. In this sense, the fact that the agency made provision for such a survey to be performed is an act of not inconsiderable courage and integrity.

Secondly, despite the length of the present volume, and despite the fact that it probably does represent the best single source of information on alcoholism treatment in Pennsylvania, it is not complete. Even in terms of treatment, it is important to remember that only treatment *programs* were considered. While these may well constitute the most significant aspect of treatment, they do not constitute its totality. Many patients with problems related to alcohol are dealt with by individual practitioners or within the context of other programs which were not covered by this survey (e.g. mental health clinics). Many more are dealt with in those AA groups which were not visited by the survey team. In terms of the overall problem of alcoholism, there are several aspects which were not dealt with at all, including such matters as the biochemical effects of alcohol, its medical consequences, its direct and indirect costs to the general public, the very complicated matter of dealing with the drunken driver, the issues involved in lowering the drinking age, and so forth. In order to be utterly comprehensive this would necessarily have been a much longer book. The problems raised by the interaction of society and ethanol, a rather simple chemical substance, are truly protean.

Finally, the degree to which these findings are generalizeable is not known. This is always a problem with a research study, and the informed reader will have to draw his own conclusions. The eminently informed opinion of the authors of the prefatory materials that this study may have a considerable degree of general validity (see their Forewords) happily coincides with the views of the research team. Neither the smallest nor the largest of the states, and itself a state of the very greatest internal variety, Pennsylvania may well represent a meaningful microcosm from which lessons of considerable applicability can be derived. Nor do we know of any other jurisdiction in which a comparable study has been mounted; though in this era of the information explosion such statements should always be made with caution.

Given all of these caveats, the research team would have to plead *nolo contendere* to a charge that it has failed to answer all questions about alcoholism, even in Pennsylvania. It does not view this as a dishonorable admission. Taking its cue from Gertrude Stein, it would be happy if the net result of its efforts were to be only that they allowed additional questions to be asked more precisely. Knowledge, at least in science, is built up gradually, by an incremental process. Even when illuminated by great flashes of insight, it requires that such intuitions be carefully and painstakingly tested. Eventually, a solid and proven structure will result.

The Authors
June, 1975

SECTION ONE

THE PLAN

Chapter 1

A Perspective of the Problem

> *All excess is ill, but drunkenness is of the worst sort: it spoils health, dismounts the mind, and unmans men; it reveals secrets, is quarrelsome, lascivious, impudent, dangerous and mad. In fine, he that is drunk is not a man, because he is so long void of reason, that distinguishes a man from a beast.*
>
> —William Penn
> *Some Fruits of Solitude,* 1693[1]

Introduction

To tell the story of alcohol is to tell the story of mankind. The two are so inextricably intertwined that separation is impossible. Indeed, since carbohydrate-containing fruits, grains, vegetables, and other natural products (e.g. honey) predate man, it is likely that alcohol does as well. Alcohol occurs naturally; all that is required is that fruit or grain be crushed under the hoofs of a passing herd, or that a marauding bear carelessly leave some honey exposed after his depradations. The action of ever-present, simple, and indestructible yeasts will eventually produce alcohol. Hence man was probably exposed to alcohol early in his evolutionary history. Recent biochemical studies, while proposing that the physiological mechanisms of opiate dependence represent a recent engraftment upon a pre-existing system, are reluctant to apply this conclusion to alcohol: "The same argument," writes Collier, "applies to other drugs of dependence, although it is weakened in the instance of ethanol by the possibility that evolving mammals might have been exposed to this substance."[2]

Man's initial encounter with alcohol is lost in pre-history. Modern commentators wax eloquent in imagining it:

> *For alcohol, in contrast to most of our cultural acquisitions, owes nothing to man's creative hand. It comes to us as a triumph not of human imagination but of human curiosity.*

Like fire, it is a natural phenomenon that man stumbled upon and gratefully bent to his use.[3]

Man's subsequent encounters enliven and illuminate every age. The Bible presents the humorous picture of Noah in his cups. By the Classical period an extremely sophisticated knowledge of the effects of alcohol is evident; Anacharsis, a Greek author whose dates are approximately 638-559 BC, described what in modern terms would be called a dose-response curve: "The vine bears three kinds of grapes: the first of pleasure, the second of intoxication, the third of disgust."[4] *Seneca, the Roman philosopher and statesman (4 BC—AD 65) felt that "drunkenness is nothing but voluntary madness."*[5] *The great German historian Theodor Mommsen, writing of roughly the same period of Roman history, concurred:*

That elegant world of fragrant ringlets, of fashionable mustachios and ruffles—merry as were its doings in the dance and with the harp, and early and late at the wine-cup—yet concealed in its bosom an alarming abyss of moral and economic ruin, of well or ill concealed despair, and frantic or knavish resolves.[6]

More pertinently for the purposes of the present study the English, establishers of the Commonwealth of Pennsylvania, were thoroughly familiar with alcohol in every period of their history. For example, Shakespeare's scene of the drunken porter in *Macbeth* is one of the great comic scenes in literature. Dr. Samuel Johnson and his circle, arbiters of English taste in the 18th century, considered questions related to alcohol carefully:

We discussed the question whether drinking improved conversation and benevolence. Sir Joshua (Reynolds) maintained it did. Johnson: *"No, Sir; before dinner men meet with great inequality of understanding; and those who are conscious of their inferiority have the modesty not to talk. When they have drunk wine every man feels himself happy, and loses that modesty, and grows imprudent and vociferous: but he is not improved: he is only not sensible of his defects."*[7]

In more recent times the poet A. E. Housman sang feelingly of the virtues of man's chosen intoxicant:

Oh, many a peer of England brews
Livelier liquor than the Muse,
and malt does more than Milton can

To justify God's ways to man.
Ale, man, ale's the stuff to drink
For fellows whom it hurts to think:
Look into the pewter pot
To see the world as the world's not.
And faith, 'tis pleasant thrill 'tis past
The mischief is that 'twill not last.[8]

It would be frivolous to preface this study with a spate of literary allusions if they did not point to some important lesson. There are several here. First, the realization that alcohol has been an object of human study ever since humans have studied anything is a testament both to the age and to the complexity of the problem. For in spite of his study of alcohol, man has not yet developed a totally satisfactory approach to it. This seeming paradox may be due to a fact which the allusions demonstrate: that alcohol is deeply and thoroughly imbedded in the entire cultural context of human society. It is notoriously difficult to change attitudes or habits which have a strong cultural base. Therefore, in the search for a more rational policy for Pennsylvania one ought to proceed with a measure of respect for this ancient and quixotic substance.

Secondly, it should be recognized that alcohol is virtually alone among drugs in having such a history. Its only possible rival is tobacco; but, without going deeply into the facts of the case, alcohol appears to be relatively more important. That commonly advanced candidate for substance honors, opium and its derivatives, cannot really compete with alcohol or tobacco. Beside them it constitutes a relatively insignificant problem. There is ample reason for this. Opium does *not* occur naturally, at least in a form in which it may readily be utilized. The technology of scoring the opium seed-pod, collecting and treating the resin, and smoking it is far more complex than that of the relatively spontaneous production of alcohol. In terms of the extraction of the active ingredient alcohol has a millenium on opium. Distillation is believed to have been discovered by an Arabian alchemist named Jabir ibn Hayyan, known to the West as Geber (whence the word "gibberish" may derive) in A.D. 800.[9] It was not until 1806, more than a thousand years later, that Sertüner extracted morphine from crude opium.

The matter of alcohol versus opium will be returned to at the close of this chapter, since it does bear upon the current situation in the Commonwealth with respect to the treatment of alcoholism. In the next section, the history of alcohol in Pennsylvania will be dealt with in further detail. But as will already be apparent it cannot be exhaustively covered. To do so one would have to write virtually a complete history of the state. Rather, an attempt will be made to relate some of the more interesting and instructive aspects of the use of the drug within the state, particularly from the earlier period of our history. This will be followed by some consideration of the production, consumption, and abuse of alcoholism in the state at the present time.

Alcohol and Pennsylvania: Yesterday

Nothing could be more indicative of the close relationship between alcohol and history in Pennsylvania than the fact that, as William Penn was sailing to the New World to establish his colony, plans were laid to intercept his vessel, capture Penn and his friends, and sell them into slavery in the West Indies in return for a cargo of rum and sugar.[10] The perpetrator of this scheme was none other than that teetotalling and witch-burning Boston divine, Cotton Mather. He was probably motivated more by religious zeal than thirst. In his letter to John Higginson detailing the plot, Mather referred to the Quakers as "heretics and malignants," and to Penn as "the chief scamp"; and he gave his opinion that this deed should be done "so that the Lord may be glorified, and not mocked on the soil of this new country with the heathen worship of these people." Fortunately for Penn and his company, *Porpoise* under Master Malachai Muscott failed to intercept *Welcome* as planned, near what Mather was pleased to call "the Cape of Cod"; and a safe landing was effected. Thus began Pennsylvania.

We are informed by a later commentator that its original inhabitants were predisposed by their prior history to the drinking of alcoholic beverages:

> *The first adventurers who settled in Pennsylvania, and parts adjacent, having been generally accustomed to the use of beer or ale in Europe, were possessed of an habitual aversion to the drinking of water. They apprehended that the air of this hot climate was unhealthy, and that the water contained some noxious quality. In these opinions they were confirmed, by observing that some persons died suddenly, who had drunk freely of cold water, when oppressed with heat and fatigue; and that severe fevers and agues prevailed in the autumnal season .... Hence, through the influence of erroneous prejudices and opinions, the early settlers of the country adopted the practice which prevailed in the West Indies, and introduced the common use of rum, imported from thence, or of an inferior kind, from New England, distilled out of molasses.*[11]

It should perhaps be added that in their propensity to drink they did not therefore differ from most other colonists. "From the day in 1642 that William Bradford* confided to his journal his astonishment at the

* Governor of Massachusetts

growth of drunkenness, the use and abuse of alcoholic beverages has been an important factor in determining the characteristics of American life."[12] The drinking of alcohol was an integral part of early colonial life in America and, some have felt, not particularly problematic; a representative statement is that "in the Colonial period, drinking took place within a social system in which it was limited and controlled. Drunkenness occurred and was punished, but it was seldom frequent or widespread."[13]

Since no empirical surveys of the incidence or prevalence of alcoholism exist for this period, it is difficult to judge the accuracy of such statements. But that alcoholic beverages were part and parcel of the life at the time is well borne out by Penn himself. His country manor at Pennsbury featured a "bake and brew house" with ample provision for the manufacture of large quantities of various alcoholic beverages. Restored in 1938-39, the manor is easily reached by automobile from Philadelphia (Penn himself was the Delaware Valley's first commuter, but used the river to get to Philadelphia daily) and is located near Tullytown and the eastern terminus of the Pennsylvania Turnpike. The brewing portion of the building occupies half of the structure, is conveniently located near the kitchen door of the manor house, and possesses, among other things, a vat of sufficient capacity to astonish the casual observer. Moreover, the estate even today produces items frequently utilized in colonial times to make alcoholic beverages. There are apples (cider), pears (perry), and honey (mead), in addition to the grains needed to make beer. The Penn Family Recipe book survives and substantiates the use of these raw materials and others besides. Those who may have wondered why Philadelphians drink to this day large quantities of birch beer may find Recipe No. 99 to be interesting as well as strangely poetic:

Too Make Burtch, by a freind at the Clift in Lewis:
Bore a hole through a burtch tree and
putt in a faset,
and putt sumthing under,
and when tis full boyle it of every 2 days
with 2 pound of white sugger too a gallan,
and when it is almost Cold,
work it up with a Littel yeist,
then put it up in Veselles
obsarve that the time to sane it is in March
and at the beginning of Aprill
if it be a forward spring it will scarse Run
at all Aprill.[14]

Nor was Penn's taste for alcoholic beverages unusual. In 1685, only three years after the bungled interception by Cotton Mather, correspondence suggests not only that his fellow colonists shared his penchant for drink but that commercial brewing had already begun in Philadelphia:

> *Our DRINK has been* Beer *and* Punch, *made of* Rum *and* water: *our Beer was mostly made of Molasses, which well boyld, with* Sassafrass *or* Pine *infused into it, makes very tolerable drink, but now they make* Mault, *and Mault drink begins to be common, especially at the* Ordinaries *and the Houses of the more substantial People. In our great Town there is an* able man, *that has set up a large* Brew House, *in order to furnish the People with Good Drink, both there and up and down the River.*[15]

If this rather idyllic picture of a general and relatively carefree consumption of alcohol was indeed accurate it was, by general agreement, not of very long life. The 18th century was "not many years old," according to Krout, "when a change came over colonial drinking customs. It was caused largely by the increasing popularity of distilled spirits in general, and rum in particular."[16] Anthony Benezet, a Quaker of French origins known principally for his active opposition to slavery, observed that by 1728 "the introduction and consumption of rum had made an amazing progress, and began to rouse the attention of some of the considerate, may I not say, of the lovers of the country in that day."[17] By balancing the imports and exports of rum as reported in the *Pennsylvania Gazette* for that year he calculated the yearly consumption of rum in the state at 25,000 pounds. Indeed, as early as 1721 the Philadelphia Friends had encouraged a movement to prevent the sale of "ardent spirits" in the province and to encourage the brewing of beer as a substitute.[18] And by 1744 a Philadelphia Grand Jury whose foreman was Benjamin Franklin presented a report deploring the existence of more than 100 public houses in the city "and representing that the court exercise more freely its power of suppression."[19]

Despite these alarms and excursions, drinking in Pennsylvania apparently flourished in an uninhibited and almost exotic manner. The die was cast early. From Colonial times to the present, the pattern has been one of continued and increased drinking, and increasingly strident efforts to stop it, culminating in the great experiment of Prohibition and its failure. To date all measures designed to abate the use of alcohol have been generally ineffective. This may be seen from a description of drinking in Pennsylvania as of 1750-54, the exact middle of the 18th century. The writer is an ingenuous German observer, Gottlieb Mittelberger of Enzweihingen in the duchy of Wurttemberg, Germany. It fell to Mittelberger's lot to accompany to America a consignment of organs which had been ordered by the famous Lutheran clergyman Henry Melchior Muhlenberg. Fortunately he recorded his impressions, and among them is a description of drinking,

18th century Pennsylvania style. Remember that this is some 30 years *after* the serious movement against spirits reported above had begun:

> *Many kinds of beverages are available in Pennsylvania and the other English colonies. First of all, excellent and salubrious water; secondly, people drink a mixture of three parts of water and one part of milk; thirdly, there is good cider; fourthly, small beer; fifth, delicious English beer, strong and sweet; sixth, so-called punch, made of three parts water and one part West Indian rum (where there is no rum, one can use brandy, but rum is much more pleasant), mixed in with sugar and lemon juice; seventh, sangaree, which is even more delicious to drink—this is made out of two parts of water and one of Spanish wine with sugar and nutmeg; and then, eighth, German and Spanish wines, which are obtainable in all taverns.*[20]

An act was passed in the Pennsylvania legislature in 1750 against "so manifest an evil," prohibiting the practice of giving out spirits on public occasions such as vendees under pain of a fine. But it also seems to have been ineffective. This may be inferred from the appearance in 1774 of a tract by Anthony Benezet. In its vehement, polemical tone the coming crusade for prohibition is clearly foreshadowed, and indeed Benezet was the spiritual father of the movement. His pupil, Dr. Benjamin Rush, was to write the most famous of all anti-alcohol pieces, and Rush's piece in turn inspired those who were the direct historical ancestors of the prohibition movement, such as Lyman Beecher of Massachusetts and the Moreau (New York) Union Temperance Society, the first temperance society in America.

Benezet's book, which was published in his hometown of Philadelphia by Joseph Crukshank, "between Second and Third Streets, in Market-Street," was entitled *The MIGHTY DESTROYER DISPLAYED, in some Account of the Dreadful Havock made by the mistaken Use as well as Abuse of DISTILLED SPIRITOUS LIQUORS, by a Lover of Mankind."* Benezet did not include all alcohol-containing beverages in his indictment, but simply those with a higher alcohol content, a lead followed by his pupil Benjamin Rush. Recent research[21] has implicated *all* classes of alcoholic beverages in alcoholism, and in fact has suggested that wine rather than distilled spirits may be the most common tipple of alcoholics,[22] though this may not have been the case a century ago.

The intensity of Benezet's feeling cannot be overstated. He described the drinking of distilled liquors as

> *An evil so amazingly great, that did not woeful experience*

too fully prove it, it seems incredible, that any whom it concerns could possibly be so negligent, as not to use their utmost endeavors to suppress this destructive manbane.[23]

Much of the pamphlet is given to various descriptions of physical problems allegedly due to alcohol which were extracted from English medical periodicals of the time. As these were not widely circulated in the colonies, Benezet felt he was performing a useful service. It is worth noting that his concern about alcohol was not unrelated to his concern about slavery. He believed that

> *... it is, in a great measure, through the introduction of these infernal spirits, that the poor Negroes have been as it were bewitched, and prevailed upon to captivate their unhappy country people, in order to bring them to the European market ...*[24]

Of particular interest is that Benezet proposed a preventive measure against the consumption of distilled spirits that has recently been revived: taxation.[25, Appendix D] Balancing the possible gains from the sale of distilled spirits against its liabilities, Benezet urged:

> *Let such lawmakers, governors, and rulers, who retain any pity for their fellow men; let these be earnestly requested seriously, and solemnly to consider, whether it is not their indispensable duty to use their utmost endeavors, that a stop may be put to this dreadful calamity; let not the apprehension of loss or any present inconveniency, deter any from doing their duty in this respect, because there cannot any inconveniences possibly arise from the redress of this grievance, which deserves to be named with those evils which will be the undoubted consequence of its continuance. The reasons which have hitherto prevailed to the countenancing of this most destructive practice ought surely to be rejected with scorn and indignation, when the welfare of such numbers are so deeply concerned. What multitudes of lives would thereby be saved, and what innumerable outrages, as theft, murder and crime prevented: To rectify which, drunkenness is made the cheapest of all vices. A device which can no otherwise be effectually prevented from raging with its present excessive enormity, and spreading devastation all around, but by laying such high taxes upon distilled spiritous liquors, as well as those made amongst us, as those imported from abroad, as will make the drinking it sufficiently expensive to put it out of the reach of so great a number of insatiable drinkers, to use it; at least in its present degree of strength.*[26]

It does not appear that Benezet's tract greatly affected his countrymen. In view of the impending Revolutionary War and its consequent upheavals, it may have gone largely unnoticed. But both Benezet's tract and his personal teachings profoundly affected one of his pupils, a man who played an important role in the Revolution as well as in American medicine. Benjamin Rush (1745-1813), who referred fondly to Benezet as "one of the most laborious schoolmasters I ever knew"[27] was a member of the Continental Congress and the only physician to be a signer of the Declaration of Independence. Edinburgh-trained, he became professor of medicine in the Philadelphia Medical College. He is considered the father of American psychiatry; his likeness adorns the seal of the American Psychiatric Association. His home in Philadelphia was restored as a project of the U.S. Bicentennial celebration, and he appeared as a character in one of the plays presented in connection with that event.

In 1785, Rush published a pamphlet whose lengthy title is reminiscent of his teacher's style: "An Inquiry into the Effects of Ardent Spirits upon the Human Body and Mind, with an Account of the Means of Preventing and of the Remedies for Curing Them." It was the first American medical treatise on alcohol, and it was enormously popular, going through many editions and being widely distributed.

If his teacher Benezet was strident about distilled spirits, Rush was apoplectic. He was hardly able to restrain himself in his detestation. Of its effects upon men he wrote:

> *In folly, it causes him to resemble a calf,—in stupidity, an ass,—in cruelty, a tyger,—in fetor, a skunk,—in filthiness, a hog,—and in obscenity, a he-goat.*

Those who may have hoped for a restrained and objective tone from a professional observer will not find it here. Nevertheless the work is not without its humor, and provides some fascinating vignettes of clinical cases of alcoholism in the Revolutionary era. A few of these are perhaps of interest here:

> *There was a citizen of Philadelphia many years ago, in whom drunkenness appeared in this protracted form. In speaking of him to one of his neighbors, I said, "Does he not* sometimes *get drunk?" "You mean," said his neighbor, "is he not* sometimes *sober?"*
>
> *I have sometimes seen (this remedy) used when a boy. In the city of Philadelphia, it was applied, by dragging the patient, when found drunk in the street, to a pump, and pumping water upon his head for 10 or 15 minutes. The*

patient generally rose, and walked off, sober and sullen, after the use of this remedy.

A citizen of Philadelphia had made many unsuccessful attempts to cure his wife of drunkenness. At length, despairing of her reformation, he purchased a hogshead of rum, and after tapping it, left the key in the door of the room in which it was placed, as if he had forgotten it. His design was to give his wife an opportunity to drink herself to death. She suspected this to be his motive, in what he had done, and suddenly left off drinking. Resentment here became the antidote to intemperance.

As merciless as was Rush toward "ardent spirits," he was nevertheless a physician who regarded the welfare of his patients above all else. Upon them he did not vent his rage, but he rather made an eloquent plea for their compassionate care. None more moving has ever appeared. A modern treatment program could do little better than to adopt as its credo what Benjamin Rush wrote a century ago:

I am aware that the efforts of science and humanity, in applying their resources to the cure of a disease introduced by an act of vice, will meet with a cold reception from many people. But let such people remember, the subjects of our remedies are their fellow creatures, and that the miseries brought upon human nature, by its crimes, are as much the objects of divine compassion (which we are bound to imitate) as the distresses which are brought upon men, by the crimes of other people, or which they bring upon themselves, by ignorance or accidents. Let us not then pass by the prostrate sufferer from strong drink, but administer to him the same relief, we would afford to a fellow creature, in a similar state, from an accidental and innocent cause.

As was the case with his teacher, Benezet, Rush's efforts did not bear immediate fruit. Palmer, an Englishman who visited Philadelphia in 1818, five years after Rush's death, remarked upon the great variety of taverns and tavern-boards there:

We observed several curious tavern signs in Philadelphia and on the roadside, among others Noah's Ark; a variety of Apostles, Bunyan's Pilgram; a cock on a lion's back, crowing, with Liberty issuing from his beak; naval engagements in which the British are in a desperate situation; the most common signs are eagles, heads of public characters, Indian Kings &c.[28]

But Rush had lighted a torch. It was not for nothing that he was dubbed by latter-day temperance workers "The True Instaurator," or inaugurator, of their movement. His work was to reach fruition more than a century from the time he originally wrote, and when the character of the country had changed considerably. But that the country had begun to change during his lifetime is clear from another notable Pennsylvania event which occurred less than a decade after the first edition of his pamphlet appeared: the Whiskey Rebellion.

One of the major attractions at Walt Disney World in Orlando, Florida, is the Hall of Presidents. It is located in a structure whose facade is an attempt to replicate Philadelphia's Independence Hall. Within the Hall the principal attraction consists in the animated effigies of all the Presidents of the United States, who speak and gesture in a lifelike manner. They are under the general direction, it would appear, of President Lincoln. Critics have scoffed at the alleged superpatriotism which they feel underlies such an exhibit. But to one observer, at least, the results were impressive; and the effect upon children is remarkable.

Following the brief animated presentation a rather more lengthy and detailed film is shown which has to do with the history of the Republic. It is this film which is significant for our present purpose. For after the initial discussion of the Revolutionary War and the events related to it, the subsequent story of the United States unfolds. The very first chapter in that story is the Pennsylvania Whiskey Rebellion. Adults of the present generation will not recall this sequence from their course of instruction in American History; but that is because only very recent events have called attention to this episode as one of great significance, as indeed it was viewed at the time. The intervention of armed federal troops at Central High School in Little Rock and at the University of Alabama had its direct precursor in events in Pennsylvania at the close of the 18th century. Because of their importance and their connection with alcohol, these events will be briefly recounted.

Although it had been victoriously prosecuted, the War of Independence had not been inexpensive. When it was over the newly united states were in desperate need of financial resources. Under the leadership of secretary of the treasury Alexander Hamilton a search was therefore made for revenue. In the Spring of 1791 the congress enacted Mr. Hamilton's proposals. They included duties upon imports and an excise tax upon certain products, prominent among which were distilled spirits (there is no direct evidence that Hamilton was influenced in this action by Benezet and Rush, though that is not impossible).

The new whiskey tax fell heavily upon western Pennsylvania. "Pennsylvania was the banner state, and western Pennsylvania the banner section, in this industry."[29] Interestingly the reasons for this had to do more with transportation problems than with the desire to consume distilled spirits. The Pennsylvania mountains were at that time a serious impediment:

> *The rich region raised grain greatly in excess of the needs of its inhabitants, but it cost more to transport a barrel of flour over the mountains than it would sell for in the markets of the east. So it was with the fruits of the region. But when these were distilled into spirits, they could be transported more readily, and sold at a profit. A horse could pack but four bushels of grain, but it could easily transport the product of 24 bushels in the form of distilled liquor.*[30]

Given these circumstances alone, it is not surprising that there was great opposition to the new tax in western Pennsylvania. But there were additional and contributory reasons for the opposition of the populace. Many were of Scotch-Irish extraction, and had a history of past resistance to taxation. The French Revolution had just begun; its anti-governmental ideology added fuel to the fires. The several border wars which had been fought in the area had given to the inhabitants a character of independence and self-determination quite apart from that of other regions. These were the frontiersmen of their day. In fact, there had been secessionist sentiment in this area before. Many people felt more loyalty to Virginia than to Pennsylvania and resented their land being considered a part of the latter state. Finally, on account of the relative remoteness of the country, it was believed unlikely that the new excise provisions could be effectively enforced by a distant federal government.

When some of the region's more responsible leaders such as Albert Gallatin* joined the opposition, the fat was in the fire. They were joined by less levelheaded and more demagogic leaders like David Bradford, a lawyer of some renown and a deputy attorney general of the state. There was increasing agitation. When attempts were finally made to collect the revenue, people turned violently upon the collectors. Several were tarred and feathered, and their homes were destroyed. A secret terrorist organization under the symbolic leadership of one "Tom the Tinker" sprang up. "A distiller who had the hardihood to go counter to the prevailing sentiment and entered his still for taxation, found a notice posted up in the night at his door, warning him that unless he aligned himself with the opposers of the excise, "Tom the Tinker" would pay him a visit and mend his still! [31]

When the federal congress responded to this pressure by modifying and abating its demands, the determination of the people of the region

* Whose statue stands in front of the U.S. Treasury Building in Washington, D.C.

to resist was greatly strengthened. President Washington finally issued a proclamation that the excise provisions would be enforced and warned all persons not to interfere. General John Neville was appointed inspector of the excise for the area. By the time he was able to mount a determined effort to collect the taxes, toward the middle of 1794, feelings were running extremely high. The spark which lit the conflagration occurred in July of that year when General Neville and Major Lenox, a United States marshall, served a writ on a farmer living near the border of Allegheny and Washington Counties. They were attacked on the road subsequently and shots were fired, though no one was injured.

A party of local citizens quickly gathered and, on the following morning, made an armed assault upon General Neville's home in the Chartiers valley. They were repulsed by the General's household servants and suffered at least one casualty. Regrouping on the following day they attacked the house with a force of 600. It was taken and destroyed, and the lives of its occupants were threatened; but fortunately they were aided in escaping by some less rabid members of the opposition. The next major event was a mass muster at Braddock's Field near Pittsburgh of some 7,000 opponents of the excise. This small army appeared for a while to pose a serious threat to the survival of the city of Pittsburgh. Though tragedy was eventually deflected by the good sense and strenuous exertions of levelheaded persons on both sides, it was clear that the situation had deteriorated to a point where decisive action was required.

General Washington was not one to hold back when his mind had been made up. He defined what had occurred as treason—in his words, "overt acts of levying war against the United States."[32] An army of 12,950 troops was immediately raised in Pennsylvania, Maryland, Virginia, and New Jersey. It was much better equipped and greater in size than the force he had commanded at Yorktown, and cost approximately a million dollars, a considerable sum in those days.[33] General Henry "Light Horse Harry" Lee, hero of the Revolutionary War (and father of General Robert E. Lee) was placed in charge. Other generals included the governors of Pennsylvania and New Jersey. The army was accompanied by Alexander Hamilton throughout its maneuvers. General Washington himself came out as far as Carlisle, where he personally heard a deputation from the Western region. The deputation attempted to work out a compromise. Washington would have none of it and ordered the troops on.

The effect of this massive and definitive action was overwhelming. General Daniel Morgan, a member of the staff of the army, wrote a letter home saying that "the alarm that these people have experienced is so great that they will never forget it, so far as to fly in the face of the law again.[34] Opposition melted and capitulation was complete. There were no battles. Order was restored. Fortunately the army was well commanded and its troops were successfully kept from revenging themselves upon the local population in return for the bitter and intemperate insults which had been directed at them. Collections on the tax were begun with no difficulties, and after a period of garrison duty the army was dismissed with the thanks of the government. Nor did the incident repeat itself; with the opening up of the Ohio Valley after the Indian Campaign of General Anthony Wayne, a new and better market was found for the whiskey and commerce was improved to the point where as early as 1802 the tax measure could be repealed.

Historians have differed as to whether Washington's truly massive response was justified. One suggested that "the national government showed a little weakness in making a foolish exhibit of its strength."[36] But another view, is that:

> *This action was not due to any sudden panic on the part of the great general and president, who for three years had been earnestly and patiently trying to compose the differences without resort to force, but came from his appreciation, with all the facts before him, that it was a grave crisis, requiring heroic treatment. No one who looks carefully at all the facts can well escape the conviction that the ship of state was among the breakers which had well nigh wrecked it.*[36]

Essentially the action demonstrated once and for all that the United States did have a federal government which was both willing and able to enforce its will on certain issues over that of the separate states by utilizing methods up to and including the deployment of its troops. While this principle has been tested on several occasions, most notably during the Civil War and recently during the era of civil rights activism, the early episode in Pennsylvania set the pattern for all that happened subsequently. Thus the Whiskey Rebellion occupies a niche of great significance in the history of the United States.

It is fitting that at this point the particular history of alcohol in Pennsylvania be brought to a close. With the emphatic establishment of the Union in an action related to the production of alcohol, alcohol's history passes from the local to the national scene. It becomes no longer a local matter but an important item in interstate commerce (see above), and its history is less uniquely connected with Pennsylvania or any other state than with the development of the country as a whole. Further, by this time the basic scenario with respect to alcohol has been well established. Essentially it is a continuing story of the increased use of, and increased opposition to the use of, alcohol in its many forms, culminating in Prohibition. It is a national, not a local story, and is one which has been well told on more than one occasion.[37,38] As for the aftermath of Prohibition—that is, the continuing attempt of a small group of states to exercise restraint over the sale of alcohol by a variety of means—Pennsylvania played an important role here, setting up the first of the state monopoly systems. While this has been and continues to be a matter of considerable controversy, it is the subject of a special report (Appendix D) and will not be further discussed.

It may be useful now to review the production and consumption of alcohol in the Commonwealth at the present time, and then to consider briefly how the citizens of Pennsylvania have gone about dealing with those of their number who have used the drug to excess.

Alcohol and Pennsylvania: Today

Pennsylvania is both a producer and a consumer of all categories of alcoholic beverages. This is so despite many efforts which have been made to curtail these activities. A certain amount of the consumption of alcohol in Pennsylvania is excessive consumption, and those individuals who engage in this kind of consumption may be termed alcoholics. (It should be noted that, for some, this is a simplistic definition of alcoholism. The debate over the nature of alcoholism will be taken up in a subsequent chapter.) In this section an attempt will be made to approach the gross parameters of the production and consumption of alcohol as it currently exists in the Commonwealth.

For purposes of simplicity we shall consider production and consumption of the three major classes of alcoholic beverages: wine, spirits, and beer. All data are derived from the national trade publications in each of these areas: the *Wine Marketing Handbook,* the *Liquor Handbook,* and the *Brewer's Almanac.*[39,41] Production will be considered first.

Wine: Pennsylvania is not a major wine producer. Until 1968, commercial wineries were not permitted to operate in the state. In that year an act was passed which permitted limited operations. A ceiling of 50,000 gallons per winery per year was imposed. Fruit used to make the wine must be grown in Pennsylvania, and marketing opportunities are closely restricted; in the main, purchases may be made only at the site of the winery. Nevertheless, in fiscal 1973 Pennsylvania produced 37,637 gallons of still wine, ranking 17th among 26 states which produce. The leading states in this field are California, with an annual production that year of more than 284 million gallons, and New York with over 31 million gallons. With respect to sparkling wines, Pennsylvania is eighth in a field of eight producers, the leaders being California with almost 16 million gallons and New York with approximately four million. Pennsylvania's output of sparkling wine in the same period was just above 3,000 gallons.

Spirits: The Commonwealth produces a moderate amount of spirits. In fiscal 1973 a total of 329,182 tax gallons were produced, giving Pennsylvania a ranking of seventh among 10 producing states. In that same year Kentucky, the leading state, produced 71,577,674 tax gallons. Four of the 65 regular distilleries in the United States were located in Pennsylvania at that time, whereas 34 of the 65 were in Kentucky.

Beer: Pennsylvania is a major producer of beer, ranking (in 1972) seventh among all states, every one of which is a producer, including the District of Columbia. The state's total production in that year was 6,585,345 barrels (there are 31 gallons in a beer barrel). This is slightly more than a third of the production of the leading state, Wisconsin, which during that same time produced 15,587,903 barrels. However, it is of interest that in that year both states had the same number of breweries—20 each. Thus Wisconsin's advantage is that its breweries are very large, while the Keystone State is known to the brewing industry as "the home of small breweries."* Pennsylvania also treats its breweries in a kinder manner than Wisconsin. Ten years ago there were 30 breweries there as compared with 25 in Pennsylvania, so that Pennsylvania's attrition rate for breweries is only half that of Wisconsin over the decade.

Consumption Data: Pennsylvania is a low consumption state in terms of wine and spirits, but ranks fourth in the consumption of beer. It is 41st among the states in adult per capita consumption of spirits and 45th in terms of consumption per $1 million of income. It is 29th among the states in adult per capita consumption of wine and 31st in consumption per $1 million of income. The closeness of these figures suggests that income levels are not a significant determinant of the lowered consumption rates in Pennsylvania for wine and spirits. It is worth noting that the consumption of those beverages which are controlled by the state liquor monopoly in Pennsylvania (wine and spirits) is low, while the consumption of that beverage which is *not* so controlled (beer) is high.

Specific data as to the consumption of alcohol in Pennsylvania are portrayed in Table 1 and compared with national averages. While the state is below average in the consumption of wine and spirits, it is above average in beer consumption. In terms of absolute alcohol equivalents there is little in the way of overall difference between average American and Pennsylvania consumption.** The average Pennsylvanian consumes just under two gallons of absolute alcohol each year, or slightly less than the average American.

Alcoholism: At this point one might ask whether there exist data which provide an appreciation of the relative or absolute size of the

* It is perhaps worth noting here that John Wagner of Philadelphia brewed the first lager beer in the United States in 1840.[42]

** The difference, which amounts to .16 gallons of absolute alcohol, would not sustain an alcoholic for four days.

TABLE I

Consumption of Alcohol in Pennsylvania

	Average Annual per capita Consumption, Gallons*			Absolute Annual Alcohol Equivalents in ml per capita	
Beverage	United States	Alcohol Pennsylvania	Assumed Absolute Content**	United States	Pennsylvania
Beer	19.10	21.40	5%	3,371.62	4,047.00
Wine	1.61	1.12	16%	975.10	675.13
Spirits	1.92	1.44	40%	2,667.04	2,180.34
				7,013.76	6,902.47

problem of alcoholism in Pennsylvania. The overall answer seems to be that some general indication can be given in both categories, but that all such figures need to be seriously qualified. Figures on the absolute incidence of alcoholism are difficult to interpret because there are problems in both the direct and the indirect measurement of alcoholism and, beyond this, in obtaining agreement on the nature of alcoholism. Figures on the relative incidence of alcoholism are difficult to interpret because the same measures are rarely utilized to measure alcoholism in different jurisdictions. Technical details of these arguments will be covered in a subsequent chapter. Here the data which are available will be summarized.

There have been two major attempts recently to estimate the overall number of alcoholics in Pennsylvania. The first of these is contained in the Pennsylvania State Alcohol Abuse and Alcoholism Plan for 1971-72.[43] The estimate is based on reported deaths due to cirrhosis of the liver and utilizes the Brenner modification of Jellinek's formula. Based on 1,812.5 average annual deaths from cirrhosis in the period 1969-70 for the entire state, it is estimated that there were in that period 944,011 alcoholics in Pennsylvania. Other ways of expressing this figure are that 8% of the overall state population or 11% of its adult population suffered from alcoholism.

A second major attempt at estimation was based on a survey done in the Spring of 1973. Using criteria related to the consumption of alcohol,

* Sources for these data are: *The Liquor Handbook*, 1973; *The Wine Marketing Handbook*, 1974; and *The Brewer's Almanac*, 1973.

** These figures are suggested by the Addiction Research Foundation of Toronto in their publication *Proposal for a Comprehensive Health Oriented Alcohol Control Policy in Ontario*, April 1973, p. 1 of Appendix 1.

Schaps and Rubin[44] estimated that there were 631,508 abusers of alcohol, or that 7.3% of the adult population were abusing alcohol. The survey data also permitted a calculation of the drinking population, in that 21.8% of the survey population indicated they did not drink at all. Hence it could be estimated that there were 6,726,169 drinkers in Pennsylvania among the adult population, and that there was roughly one alcoholic for every 10 persons who drank at all.

Beyond noting that the ranges do not differ greatly between the two studies there is no real way to decide between them. Hence we can say only that there may be between 6.32×10^5 and 9.44×10^5 alcoholics, or that between 7.3% and 11% of the adult population are alcoholics. Just how this compares with other states is quite problematic. However, one may note that a careful national sample[45] revealed an incidence among adults of 9%, a figure which is almost exactly in the middle of our two most recent estimates. Since Pennsylvanians approach the national average in terms of the consumption of absolute alcohol (see Table 1), and there is evidence[46] of a linear relationship between consumption of alcohol and alcoholism, it is tempting to conclude that Pennsylvania is probably at the national average in terms of the number of alcoholics per 100,000 citizens. Until there are considerable improvements in the ability of both Pennsylvania and the nation at large to measure the incidence and prevalence of alcoholism, both cross-sectionally and longitudinally over time (something which seems a necessary prelude to any rational alcohol policy), such a statement may serve as the best we can do at the moment. Certainly any problem which affects hundreds of thousands of Pennsylvanians merits only the most serious attention.

The Treatment of Alcoholism in Pennsylvania—Yesterday (1840-1959)

But what sort of attention has the problem received? For a number of reasons, this is not an easy question to answer. Much of the effort put forth over the years to assist the alcoholic has gone unreported. Many individuals, among them physicians, clergymen, and numerous lay people, have contributed but have not recorded their work. They have failed to do so partly out of modesty. In addition, they have seen the assistance which they rendered not as a particular type of help given to an individual with a particular type of problem, but as merely a part of their general helping effort, whether it be to save bodies or to save souls. There has not emerged a separate and distinct alcoholism treatment effort. Rather (for the most part) assistance to the alcoholic has been rendered as a part of general assistance to the ill and needy, at least until recently.

Hence it is difficult to do justice to all who have played a role in the process. What follows is necessarily incomplete and does not give sufficient credit to many. Regrettable as this may be, it is nevertheless useful to bear in mind, for it anticipates the major conclusion of this study: that society has not yet come to grips with the problem of alcoholism in any systematic manner, and a systematic record of the alcoholism treatment effort does not exist. An attempt will be made in this chapter to sketch what has been done in the past and the remainder of the work will describe the situation at present in the Commonwealth. But the limitations of both aspects of the study should not be overlooked.

As nearly as can be determined, the notion that alcoholics constitute a group of people who ought to be helped is relatively recent. Not until the founding of the Washingtonian Movement in 1840 was any large-scale effort made, and this despite the fact that the temperance movement had begun some time before. The temperance movement was preventive, not therapeutic. It was designed to keep people from succumbing to the vice of alcoholism, not to rescue them from it once they had "fallen." Dr. Harrison in 1860 attributed this in part to a class bias in the temperance movement, noting that "our temperance friends were, generally, men in higher circles of life, who would revolt at the idea of taking a drunkard by the arm in the street and walk with him in some place where he could be made sober and receive friendly advice."[47] Milton Maxwell has summed up the situation quite well:

> *As for the alcoholic, it was the prevailing opinion, up to 1840, that nothing could be done to help him. Occasionally a "drunkard" did "reform," but this did not erase the general pessimism as to the possibility of rehabilitating drunkards. Since alcohol was held to be the "cause" of alcoholism, the temperance movement was aimed solely at keeping the non-alcoholic from becoming an alcoholic. This implied indifference to the alcoholic was epitomized by Justin Edwards in 1822: "Keep the temperate people temperate; the drunkards will soon die, and the land be free."*[48]

This unfortunate situation was altered, however briefly, by the formation and propagation of a remarkable organization known as the Washingtonian Society. Arising from the efforts of a group of drinking cronies in a Baltimore Tavern in April, 1840, the Society was essentially a self-help movement among the afflicted. In that sense it was an earlier precursor of Alcoholics Anonymous, though the historical connections between the two movements are in reality rather tenuous. AA seems mainly to have learned from the mistakes of the former effort (see Chapter 13). Somehow, the Washingtonian idea took hold. Propelled by several charismatic individuals and spellbinding orators, such as John Gough, the movement had an almost incredible vogue for a few brief years, though it was essentially over by 1848.

As is the case with many other self-help movements, the Washingtonian Movement resembled an evangelical and religious effort.[49] Mass meetings were held at which former drunkards recounted the almost miraculous tale of their reformation, aided by the brethren of the Society, and urged others to come forward and be helped. "No fiction could be more exciting or dramatic. These true-life narratives pulled at the heartstrings. They aroused awe and wonder at the 'miracle of rebirth'."[50] In June of 1841 the team of Jesse Vickers and Jesse W. Small began a campaign in Pittsburgh, where " 'all classes, all ages, all ranks and denominations, and both sexes, presses every night into overflowing churches.' In a brief time, 10,000 were pledged, 'including a multitude of the most hopeless characters.'."[51] Both Philadelphia and Pittsburgh were considered centres of the movement, and it was estimated that in and around Philadelphia (where for some reason the societies were called Jeffersonian rather than Washingtonian) some 20,000 members were enrolled.

The fervor did not last long. While the Washingtonians were initially useful to the temperance movement, they became something of an embarrassment when the novelty wore off, especially as some of their more prominent spokesmen regressed to the bottle. Moreover, they eschewed the political and legalistic maneuvers which began to appeal increasingly to the temperance movement and were to become their eventual means of triumph (Prohibition was essentially a tribute to the astute politicking of Wayne B. Wheeler, the formidable General Counsel of the Anti-Saloon League).[53] Finally, like many evangelical movements, the participants fell to bickering among themselves and split into factions. In essence, the movement burned itself out. Small remnants survived; there is yet a Washingtonian Institution in Boston, now newly revived and effectively functioning. But the history of the Washingtonian Movement serves principally to illustrate the fact that little was being done to help alcoholics in mid-19th century America.

A generation later, in the period of the 1870s, there appeared an association of lay and professional people who had become convinced that alcoholism was a special problem and required special treatment, and who set about to provide the same. The American Association for the Cure of Inebriates was a loose confederacy of institutions and individuals. Its origins were apparently multi-focal; for example, the Pennsylvania Sanitarium at Media had been founded some time before, in 1866. Joseph Parrish, M.D., its director, scion of a proud Philadelphia medical family (and ancestor of the late great artist Maxfield Parrish), became president of the Association and was one of its leading lights. By 1874 the Association listed nine institutions as members. They included the Washingtonian Homes in Boston and Chicago and the New York State Inebriate Asylum at Binghampton. Two institutional members are listed for Pennsylvania: the Franklin Reformatory Home for Inebriates at 913-15 Locust Street in Philadelphia, and the Inebriate Department of the House of Corrections, also in Philadelphia. (The Media Sanitarium is not listed in 1874 and

Parrish appears in the rolls of that year as the Superintendent of Harlem Lodge in Baltimore; apparently the institution had folded.)[54]

The major thrust of the Association was to promote separate treatment for alcoholics. In his Presidential Address of September 28, 1875, Joseph Parrish reported with evident satisfaction that the Superintendents of Hospitals for the Insane, at their recent annual meeting, had come out for separate inebriate institutions "for the reason, that the presence of inebriates in the hospitals under their charge, is injurious to the insane."[55] While it was understandable that the superintendents should feel this way, Parrish was more concerned for his own. In the instructions to patients at Media appeared the following: "You are not insane, and do not require the restraints of insanity. You are morally infirm, and need self-discipline and culture. You are physically diseased, and need medical treatment."[56]

At least on a temporary basis the Association met with some success. Some of its institutions were fairly substantial. In an 1871 report Media claimed 186 admissions for "alcoholic inebriety" and 14 admissions for "opium inebriety."[57] The Franklin Reformatory Home reported 112 admissions and 44 re-admissions during its first year of operation.[58] A typical case summary from the Superintendent's Report of the Franklin Reformatory Home, April 1, 1873 may be of interest. We are now roughly a century from the reports of Dr. Rush and another century from our own era:

> *Mr. ______ was a young man who commenced drinking in the Army. He was genial and social in his habits, and this one became so fixed that he was declared a hopeless case. He would absent himself from home and wander over the city, drinking constantly. He was brought to us in a state of* mania-potu *just after the House was opened, before organization was complete, and was removed before any moral influences could be brought to bear upon him. In three months he again fell, and a member of the Godwin Association hearing of it, had him brought back by the Association in a terrible condition. He was carefully nursed and cared for, and his attention fully aroused to the fact that he had nearly added his name to the list of victims of this fearful vice. He became an earnest reformed man, and is, and has been since July, a sober man, a consolation to his parents, and one of the most faithful and efficient workers in the Association.*[59]

(The Godwin Association was an organization of the graduates of the Franklin Reformatory Home, who assisted each other subsequent to their recovery. Hence the self-help impulse was still very active despite the passing of the Washingtonians.)

While the eventual fate of the American Association for the Cure of Inebriates is not known, it can be said that, if it did not survive as a group and failed to achieve any ultimate success in the establishment of separate treatment facilities, it nevertheless helped to keep that issue alive. Indeed in 1903 the Commonwealth of Pennsylvania passed an Inebriate Act which called for the commitment of a drunkard "to a proper hospital, or asylum, for restraint, care, and treatment."[60] Little was done, however; and in January of 1908 Dr. John Beans Carrell, a physician of Hatboro and a member of the Inebriate Hospital Committee of the State Medical Society, read a paper before the Philadelphia County Medical Society in complaint. No facility yet existed, and the inebriate was treated as either a criminal or insane. Dr. R. H. Chase of the Friend's Asylum for the Insane in Frankford is recorded as making the following statement, reminiscent of those in the 1870s:

> *The institutions for the insane are not well adapted for the care and treatment of this class. The alcoholic resents as an insult his enforced association with the insane, and on the other hand the self-respecting insane person feels affronted that through the exigency of his misfortune he should be made to affiliate with members of a class whom he had hitherto regarded with more or less contempt. The mixture of the two elements seems to be as incompatible as the most rebellious chemical ingredients.*[61]

In spite of the weight of this and other opinions and the sincere efforts of many persons to secure facilities for inebriates, once again little movement was evident. This was not merely the case in Pennsylvania. In 1917 Horatio Pollock and Edith Furbush surveyed the institutional management of inebriates and others in the United States for the National Committee for Mental Hygiene. They found[62]

TABLE 2

Institutional Care in the United States and in Pennsylvania on January 1, 1917. Data Are from Pollock and Furbush (61).

	Number in Institutions	
Class of Individual	United States	Pennsylvania
Insane	234,055	19,436
Feebleminded	37,220	4,361
Epileptics	10,801	645
Inebriates	4,891	429

that there were 571 institutions in the country as of January 1, 1917 for the management of the insane, the feebleminded, epileptics, and inebriates. Of these there were but four state institutions (Connecticut, Iowa, Massachusetts, and Minnesota) and 28 private institutions for inebriates only.

Their census showed that a total of 4,891 inebriates were receiving institutional care in the United States at that time. This was, by a very substantial margin, the smallest of all of the four categories which were considered (see Table 2). Of the overall figure, 3,991, inebriates were in public institutions and 900 were in private institutions. The authors commented specifically that "the extent of private care of inebriates is also very meager. In New Jersey 203 cases were reported in private institutions; in every other state the number was less than 100."

Such was the general situation on the eve of World War I. With respect to Pennsylvania, at least, there is little evidence that much of significance was done regarding the public care of the alcoholic until after World War II. This does not mean that nothing whatever was done; many individuals no doubt put forth a sincere and determined effort, and it is regrettable that there is no way of acknowledging our particular debt to them. This period also saw the founding (1935) and rise of that remarkable organization, Alcoholics Anonymous, by all odds the single most important effort in the alcoholism treatment field ever mounted (see Chapter 11). Nevertheless, the impression remains of a lack of substantial and organized effort, particularly of public and governmental effort.

A notable exception of this was Dr. Charles Dudley Saul (1880-1947), medical director of Saint Luke's and Children's Medical Center of Philadelphia from 1941 until his death. Dr. Saul had begun to treat alcoholism at the hospital as early as 1938. As a result, we are told (in a statement reminiscent of Drs. Parrish, Carrell, and others) that

> *. . . he became convinced that the individualistic method was not adequate and began to plan a clinic where alcoholics might be separated from other sick people and given an opportunity to learn about their disease by discussion with fellow sufferers. The advent of the war, however, blocked any development of this plan until 1946.*[63]

The Saul Clinic finally opened on June 10, 1946, shortly before Dr. Saul's death. It was named in honor of the man "who boldly called our profession's attention to its responsibility in the treatment of alcoholism and stimulated the interest of physicians and psychiatrists."[64] The basic idea of the clinic, as described by its first medical superintendent, was to "give these individuals a sober moment to analyze their problem so that they can decide what they wish to do about it."[65] Hence, short-term rather than long-term hospital treatment

TABLE 3

Estimated Number of Substance Abusers per 10,000 Adults, by Geographic Strata, Pennsylvania, 1973. Calculated from Reference (43).

	per 10,000 adults:	
Stratum	Est. No. Opiate Abusers	Est. No. Alcohol Abusers
Urban Counties	120	920
Suburban Counties	100	630
Small Cities	80	750
Rural Counties	70	540
Pennsylvania	92	734

was stressed; in addition, there was a heavy emphasis upon medical management as well as interaction with Alcoholics Anonymous. Thirty-three patients were admitted in June and 48 in July,[66] while the total count between the opening of the unit and April 30, 1949 was 2,878 admissions.[67] Obviously, the Saul Clinic was a going concern. It still is, and is one of the treatment programs included in the major portion of this report.

Unfortunately, however, it stood alone at the time. In the year after the clinic was founded, a resolution was passed by the General Assembly of the Commonwealth directing the Joint State Government Commission to investigate the problem of alcoholism in Pennsylvania. A subcommittee was appointed which reviewed the existing literature, held a hearing, and visited the Saul Clinic. Despite the fact that there may have been as many as 58,000 alcoholics in Pennsylvania at that time, the only action which the state legislature had thus far taken was to provide $50,000 over a two-year period for the Saul Clinic. The Committee recommended that the biennial appropriation be continued and matched with a similar appropriation for Pittsburgh. The Department of Health was asked to develop a better statistical estimate of alcoholism. In an interesting turn of phrase it was "deemed inexpedient" to require medical and nursing schools to teach courses concerning alcoholism, though they were encouraged to do so. Likewise, hospitals were "encouraged" to admit alcoholics. In sum, it is rather a dreary record and the lack of legislative enthusiasm is all too evident.[68]

With the advent of the Saul Clinic, a participant in our current study, we have almost arrived in the present. Yet it is useful to look at a document which appeared in 1959, some 13 years later. *The Alcoholism Handbook and Directory of Facilities,* published by the Department of

TABLE 4

Ratio of Available Treatment Slots to Number of Estimated Abusers, Pennsylvania, 1973. Calculated from Reference (43).

	Treatment Slots Available for:	
Stratum	Opiate Abusers	Alcohol Abusers
Urban Counties	1: 7.6	1: 43.8
Suburban Counties	1: 9.1	1: 57.5
Small Cities	1:26.9	1:225.4
Rural Counties	1:77.1	1:155.2
Pennsylvania	1: 9.6	1:102.4

Public Health of the City of Philadelphia, listed all facilities in the five-county area of southeast Pennsylvania which were in use at the time for the treatment of alcoholism. Under the rubric "medical facilities primarily for alcoholism" we may find the sort of institutions under consideration here. At that time there were but five: the Malvern Institute, the Saul Clinic, Willow Grove Hospital, the Alcoholism Control Unit, an out-patient operation at 415 West Girard, and the Philadelphia Counseling Center for Alcoholism at 915 Corinthian. While some improvement in services had obviously occurred, the overall effort remained unimpressive, especially in view of the size of the population of the five-county area.[69]

In more recent times an increased effort has been mounted in Pennsylvania to deal with the problem of the treatment of alcoholism. The major purpose of this report is to survey and assess that effort, and the results are reported in the chapters that follow. It will be seen that, while much has been done, much remains to do. In addition to the many factors which have contributed to a lack of progress in the past, there is an entirely new factor impinging upon the development of alcoholism treatment. This is the impact of the treatment being provided to opiate abusers. It has not been important previously because the scope of the narcotic addiction treatment effort was minimal. But it now appears to be a factor of some significance and will be briefly considered. A more detailed presentation appears in a separate publication.[70]

There can be little question that alcoholism is more prevalent than narcotic addiction. Table 3 presents data drawn from the Schaps and Rubin study, which considered both problems. It shows that in Pennsylvania as a whole, as well as in each geographic stratum of the state, alcoholism is far more common. Now, if this were a strictly rational world, it would follow that treatment facilities would be provided according to the number of persons who suffer from an illness. Such is not the case. Table 4, taken from the same study, shows that exactly the opposite is true. Roughly speaking, there is one treatment slot for every 10 narcotic addicts and only one slot for every 100 alcoholics, in spite of the fact that there are about eight times as many alcoholics as addicts.

Thus in the field of addiction treatment we have a paradox. Less treatment is available for the larger problem. It is not unique to this field.[71] But it may be due to a unique cause. This is suggested by a graph (Figure 1) showing the establishment dates of alcoholism treatment programs considered in this study and comparing them with the establishment dates of narcotic addiction treatment programs considered in a previous study.[72] The graph shows that, as the establishment of narcotic addiction treatment programs increased in the period after 1965, the establishment of alcoholism treatment programs decreased. The data suggest—though they do not prove—that there may be a causal relationship between these two phenomena. A version of Gresham's Law may be operative in the addiction field. Treatment for narcotic addiction may tend to drive out treatment for alcoholism. Perhaps the converse is true as well. There are many possible explanations for this phenomenon but, in this age of inflation, the most persuasive may be the economic. A finite amount of capital is available for the treatment effort in both fields; hence, when one aspect captures the popular imagination it is differentially subsidized, and the other aspect suffers.

Logically, of course, this is unfortunate. Problems ought to be dealt with according to a rational ordering of priorities. This does not appear to be happening in the addiction field. With the advent of single state and federal agencies devoted to the addictions, and with the dawning of the belief that all citizens have a right to treatment for their health problems, including drug and alcohol abuse, there may finally come a time when there is an equitable distribution of treatment capability. But the historical odds against such an eventuality are obviously quite high.

In summary, mankind in general and Pennsylvanians in particular have had a long and troubled relationship with alcohol. They have also had a long and troublesome record of *not* providing adequately for problems due to alcoholism, even though the need for this has been clearly and consistently seen by at least a portion of the citizenry. Recently, the added problem of dealing with a similar difficulty, narcotic addiction, may have had an adverse effect upon the overall alcoholism treatment effort. The following report will suggest that, despite many admirable attempts, the goal of adequate service has not yet been reached.

FIGURE 1

ESTABLISHMENT DATE OF DRUG AND ALCOHOL PROGRAMS IN PENNSYLVANIA

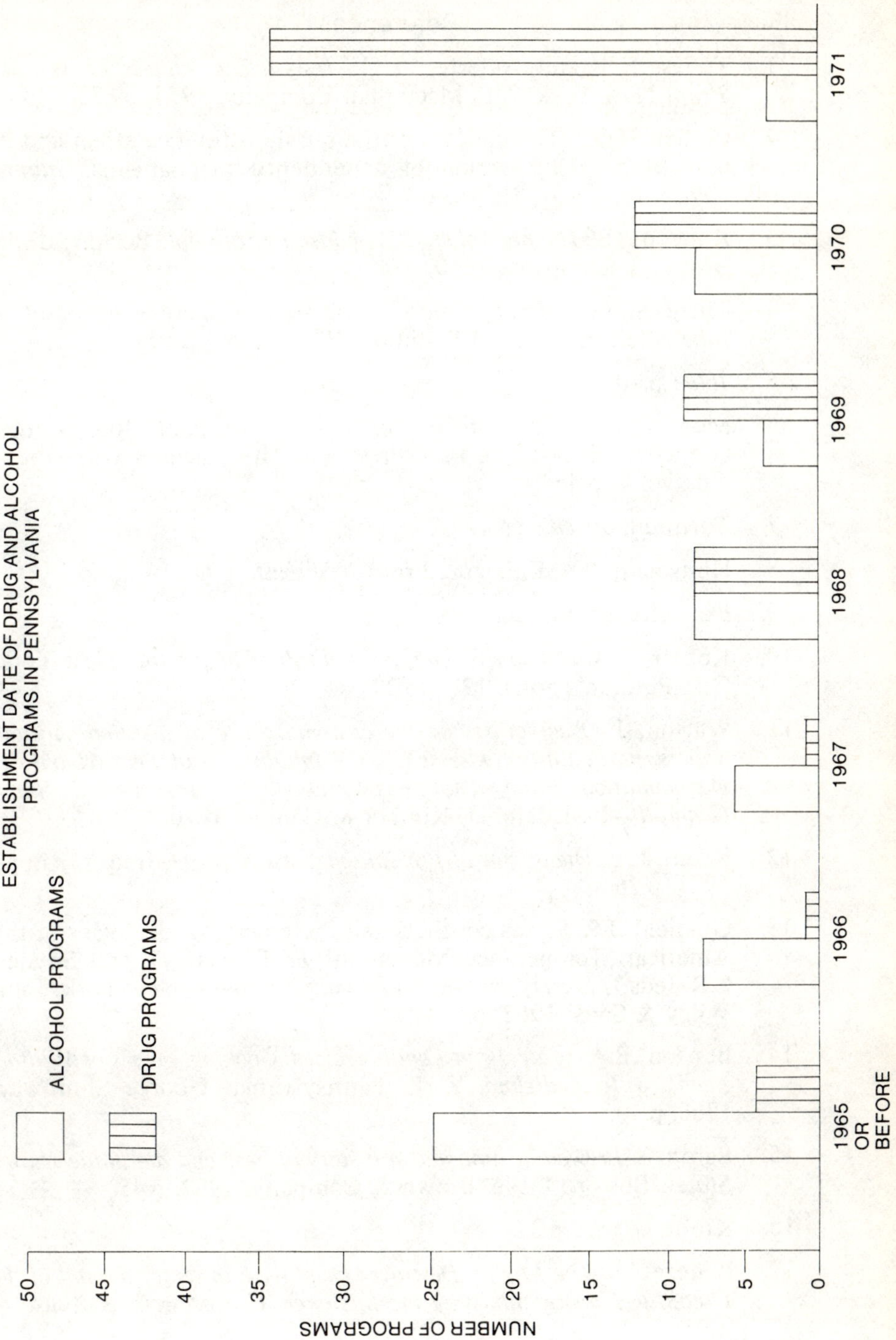

References

1. Tolles, F.B. and Alderfer, E.G., (eds.). *The witness of William Penn.* New York: The Macmillan Company, 1957, p.173.
2. Collier, H.O.J. The concept of the quasi-abstinence effect and its use in the investigation of dependence mechanisms. *Pharmacology, 11:* 58-61, 1974.
3. Roueche, B. *The neutral spirit: A portrait of alcohol.* Boston: Little, Brown & Company, 1960, p. 4.
4. Turnbull, G.H. *Fruit of the vine: As seen by many witnesses of all times.* Baltimore: Lord Baltimore Press, 1951, p.103.
5. *Ibid.,* p.107.
6. Mommsen, T. *The history of Rome.* Translator Anonymous. Glencoe, Illinois: The Free Press and The Falcon's Wing Press. n.d., vol *4,* p.464.
7. Turnbull, *op. cit.,* pp.123-24.
8. Housman, A.E. Epilogue. From *A Shropshire lad.*
9. Roueche, *op. cit.,* p.21.
10. Kobler, J. *Ardent spirits: The rise and fall of Prohibition.* New York: G.P. Putnam's Sons, 1973, p.29.
11. Watson, J. *Observations on the customary use of distilled spiritous liquors, particularly addressed to the Inhabitants of Pennsylvania of Denominations, and also to the People of the United States Generally.* Philadelphia: Kimber & Conrad, 1810.
12. Krout, J.A. *The origins of Prohibition.* New York: Alfred A. Knopf, 1925, p.26.
13. Gusfield, J.R. Status conflicts and the changing ideologies of the American Temperance Movement. *In:* Pittman, J. and Snyder, C.R. (eds.): *Society, culture, and drinking patterns.* New York: John Wiley & Sons, 1962, p.104.
14. Benson, E.A. (ed.). *Penn Family recipes: Cooking recipes of William Penn's wife Gulielma.* York, Pennsylvania: George Shumway, 1966, p.40.
15. Baron, S. *Brewed in America: A history of beer and ale in the United States.* Boston: Little, Brown & Company, 1962, p.45.
16. Krout, *op. cit.,* p.31.
17. Benezet, A. *The Mighty Destroyer Displayed, in some Account of the Dreadful Havock made by the mistaken Use as well as Abuse of*

DISTILLED SPIRITOUS LIQUORS, by a Lover of Mankind. Philadelphia: Joseph Crukshank, 1774, p.21.

18. Krout, op. cit., p.37.

19. *Ibid.,* p.12.

20. Mittelberger, G. *Journey to Pennsylvania.* Edited and translated by O. Handlin and J. Clive. Cambridge: The Belknap Press, 1960, pp.50-51.

21. Popham, R.E., Schmidt, W., and deLint, J. The prevention of alcoholism: epidemiological studies of the effects of government control measures. Manuscript. To be published in: Ewing, J.A. and Rouse, B.A. (eds.): *Law and drinking behaviour.* Chapel Hill: University of North Carolina Press. See esp. pp.10-12.

22. Schmidt, W. and Bronetto, J. Death from liver cirrhosis and specific alcoholic beverage consumption: an ecological study. *American Journal Public Health,* 52: 1473-82 (Sept.) 1962.

23. Benezet, *op. cit.,* p.4.

24. *Ibid.,* p.12.

25. Popham et al., *op. cit.*

26. Benezet, *op. cit.,* pp.43-44.

27. Rush, B. *An inquiry into the effects of ardent spirits upon the human body and mind, with an account of the means of preventing and the remedies for curing them.* First published in 1785. Brookfield: E. Merriam & Company, 1814 (Eighth Edition). Reprinted in the *Journal of Studies on Alcohol, 4:* 321-41, September 1943.

28. Brown, J.H. *Early American beverages.* Rutland: Charles E. Tuttle, 1966, p.140.

29. Cutler, W.G. The nation's first rebellion. *Magazine of American History. 12:* 332-47, 1884, p.334.

30. Wiley, Richard T. *The whiskey insurrection: A general view.* Elizabeth, Pennsylvania: Herald Printing House, 1912, p.15.

31. *Ibid.,* p.19.

32. *Ibid.,* p.30.

33. *Ibid.,* p.6.

34. *Ibid.,* p.46.

35. Cutler, *op. cit.,* p.346.

36. Wiley, *op. cit.,* p.6.

37. Kobler, *op. cit.*

38. Krout, *op. cit.*

39. *Wine Marketing Handbook.* New York: Gavin-Jobson Associates, 1974.

40. *The Liquor Handbook.* New York: Gavin-Jobson Associates, 1973.

41. *The Brewer's Almanac.* Washington: United States Brewers' Association, 1972.

42. Baron, *op. cit.,* p.176.

43. Barrett, M. *The Pennsylvania State Alcohol Abuse and Alcoholism Plan for 1971-72.* Harrisburg: Commonwealth of Pennsylvania, 1972, vol. *I,* A design for action, p.25, Exhibit I.

44. Schaps, E. and Rubin, E.L. A study of prevalence and intensity of drug and alcohol use in the Commonwealth of Pennsylvania. Harrisburg: Governor's Council on Drug and Alcohol Abuse, August 10, 1973.

45. Cahalan, D. *Problem drinkers.* San Francisco: Jossey-Bass, 1970, p.36.

46. deLint, J. and Schmidt, W. The epidemiology of alcoholism. *In: Biological basis of alcoholism,* ed. Y. Israel and J. Mardones, New York: Wiley, 1971, pp.423-42.

47. Maxwell, M.A. The Washingtonian Movement. *Journal of Studies on Alcohol, 11:* 410-51, 1950. p.432.

48. *Ibid.,* pp.411-12.

49. Glaser, F.B. Some historical aspects of the drug-free therapeutic community. *American Journal of Drug and Alcohol Abuse, 1:* 37-52 (May) 1974.

50. Maxwell, *op. cit.,* p.419.

51. *Ibid.,* p.421.

52. *Ibid.,* p.423.

53. Kobler, *op. cit.,* pp.180-83 ff.

54. Harris, R.P. Untitled volume of bound reports, bearing in pencil the name of Dr. R. P. Harris. Privately bound, no publisher. Library of the College of Physicians of Philadelphia, 6P/15.

55. Parrish, J. Annual Address before the American Association for the Cure of Inebriates. by J. Parrish, M.D., President, September 28, 1875.

56. Parrish, J. and 22 others. *Address to the people* by the Directors, Pennsylvania Sanitarium. Philadelphia: Henry B. Ashmead, 1871, p.15.

57. *Ibid.,* p.11.

58. Harris, *op. cit.*

59. *Ibid.*

60. Carrell, J.B. Why Pennsylvania should build, equip, and maintain a hospital for the restraint, care, and treatment of inebriates, and what the hospital should be. *Pennsylvania Medical Journal, 11:* 628-36, 1908, pp.628-69.

61. *Ibid.,* p.631.

62. Pollock, H.M., and Furbush, E.M. Insane, feebleminded, epileptics and inebriates in institutions in the United States, January 1, 1917. *Mental Hygiene,* vol. *1,* no. 4, October 1917. Pagination not given.

63. *Studies in alcoholism: A report on the work of the C. Dudley Saul clinic, 1946-49.* Published by the Board of Trustees of St. Luke's and Children's Medical Center, September 1949, p.1.

64. Davis, C.N. Experience in short term hospitalization of the alcoholic. *Journal of Studies on Alcohol, 8:* 55-60, 1947, p.55.

65. *Ibid.,* p.59.

66. *Ibid.,* pp.59-60.

67. *Studies in Alcoholism,* p.9.

68. Brunner, C.H., Jr. Alcoholism: A report of the Joint State Government Commission to the General Assembly of the Commonwealth of Pennsylvania. December 1948

69. Linden, M.E. *Alcoholism handbook and directory of facilities.* Published by the Division of Mental Health, Public Health Services, Department of Public Health, City of Philadelphia, 1959, pp.43-50.

70. Glaser, F.B., and Greenberg, S.W. Relationship between treatment facilities and prevalence of alcoholism and drug abuse. *Journal of Studies on Alcohol, 36* (3): 348-358, March 1975.

71. Kunitz, S.J. Some notes on physiologic conditions as social problems. *Social Science and Medicine, 8:* 207-11, April 1974.

72. Adler, F., Moffett, A.D., Glaser, F.B., Ball, J.C., and Horvitz, D. *A systems approach to drug abuse treatment.* Philadelphia: Dorrance and Company, 1974.

Chapter 2

Visiting the Treatment Programs

In a previous study of drug abuse treatment in the Commonwealth of Pennsylvania,[1] the survey team had begun with the assumption (based on a pilot study of programs in a major metropolitan area) that a concerted and conscious effort would be required to produce a comprehensive treatment system. While some initial steps had been taken to achieve this goal, it was felt that additional effort was needed. The outcome of the study suggested that this assumption was correct. With respect to the current study, there appeared to be no compelling reason why the situation with respect to treatment for problems related to alcohol should be any different. Accordingly, the survey team's efforts were viewed, as before, as being only the first phase of a three-phase approach which might eventually produce the desired system of treatment:

1. Identifying the existing elements of the system;
2. Assembling the system
   a. assuring that the elements to be used meet minimum standards
   b. adding whatever elements are missing
   c. connecting the elements and operationalizing the system;
3. Measuring the efficacy of the system.

As was noted in the study on the treatment of drug abuse, the tasks of Phase I took on a ready rationale when viewed from the perspective of the attempt to construct a treatment system:

> *... the first thing which must be done in establishing such a treatment system was to find out what was already being done, that is, to identify the existing treatment programs in the State ... it would be important to determine how many programs there were, and of what kind, how many persons were being treated, and of what kind, where the programs were located, and so forth. An impression could also be gained whether the programs encountered met minimal standards and whether any critical element (from a programmatic or functional viewpoint) was missing.*[2]

Relevant federal legislation mandates that such information be gathered with respect to alcoholism treatment, just as was the case with respect to treatment for drug abuse. Item 4 of subsection (a) of section 303 of Title III of Public Law 91-616, known as the "Comprehensive Alcohol Abuse and Alcoholism Prevention, Treatment, and Rehabilitation Act of 1970) (popularly called the Hughes Act in honor of its chief sponsor, Senator Harold Hughes of Iowa) provides that each state must

> *set forth ... a survey of need for the prevention and treatment of alcohol abuse and alcoholism, including a survey of the health facilities needed to provide services for alcohol abuse and alcholism and a plan for the development and distribution of such facilities and programs throughout the State. (See appendix C.)*

Such a document was prepared prior to the initiation of the present survey. Entitled *The Pennsylvania State Alcohol Abuse and Alcoholism Plan for 1971-1972,* it attempted to portray, on the basis of already existing information, the treatment situation in the Commonwealth.[3] However, the report stated that existing information was less than adequate and that a project similar to the present one would be required to provide a more satisfactory view, Thus, it noted that "in the absence of a comprehensive statewide survey, the number of facilities that serve the alcoholic and his family in Pennsylvania currently are not known."[4]

Because of the apparent similarity of the situations with respect to alcoholism and drug abuse treatment in the Commonwealth, and particularly because neither appeared to have been approached in any systematic manner prior to the time that the surveys were done, it was felt that a method of approach similar to that utilized in the drug abuse study could be used in the study of the treatment of alcoholism (see especially Chapters Two and Three of reference 1). However, some modifications were necessary at the outset because of the differing nature of the problem. Therefore a brief description of certain aspects of the methodology will be given.

What Is An Alcoholism Treatment Program?

It was necessary to develop a practical, concrete, working definition of a treatment program. The definition which was eventually used arbitrarily focused the survey on those organizational entities which were devoted exclusively to the treatment of alcohol abusers and which were treating a minimum of 10 patients at the time of contact. By "exclusive treatment" was meant that the alcoholic had to be dealt with in a programmatically different manner than those populations which were being dealt with in the same (or in a related) context. Thus, for example, if a community mental health centre numbered alcoholic persons among its clients but dealt with them in exactly the same manner as it dealt with all its other clients, it would not conform to the survey definition of a treatment program. However, as was the case in many instances, if the centre operated a separate program specifically for problem drinkers which was different in its approach from the services provided to other clients, the definition was considered fulfilled. The minimum census of 10 patients was a practical requirement to screen out programs offering services on a small-scale or irregular basis. A further requirement was that all programs visited keep separate data on the group of patients being served. In addition, there had to be at least one staff member who devoted a substantial portion of his or her time to the treatment of abusers. In other words, a functionally cohesive alcoholism treatment program had to exist. Thus, the goal of the definition was to include in the survey only those programs offering stable, ongoing treatment to alcoholics.

While it was recognized that many alcoholics receive significant service either from private individual practitioners or as an ancillary part of services intended primarily for other populations (e.g. the mentally ill), for purely practical reasons these aspects of service delivery were excluded from consideration. It would have been physically impossible to visit every family doctor, psychiatrist, hospital emergency ward, or other small-scale service providers. By delimiting the programs, we sought to include only those that were established, ongoing, relatively permanent enterprises.

What was obtained through this survey, therefore, may be summarized as a view of the institutional treatment of alcoholism in Pennsylvania in 1972-73, providing that the term "institutional" is construed in the broadest sense. As used here it implies rational organizational structure but does not necessarily mean an in-patient setting. Since there is no systematic reporting of the population of alcoholics under care in circumstances other than those covered in this survey, it is difficult to know how representative the sample was, either of programs or of clients. It is our belief that the programs examined herein constitute the major thrust of the Commonwealth's efforts against alcoholism. Certainly they represent that portion of the effort which is directly under public control and, hence, relatively amenable to change.

The Location of the Programs

One of the more difficult (and indeed vexing) problems faced by the survey team was to obtain a complete listing of all programs which potentially conformed to this definition. Perhaps more than any other aspect of the survey, the difficulties involved in this preliminary step reflected the disorganized, embryonic state of the treatment system. At the time the field work began, the single state agency which was responsible for policy-making in the area of drug and alcohol abuse was not yet involved in program operations. The responsibility for this was dispersed over several state agencies. Thus, the team had to rely on a series of incomplete and overlapping lists obtained from the various departments. In addition, several members of the team were familiar with a few of the larger programs. In order to supplement this haphazard collection, we made countless phone calls to county administrative units, relevant private agencies, religious organizations, and charitable groups. Painfully slow and frustrating as its accumulation was, the master list of probable programs provided an invaluable object lesson for the need to integrate drug and alcohol abuse treatment on the state level, an event which finally occurred.

The next step involved extensive contact with the individual treatment agencies by letter and telephone. A great deal of preliminary data were gathered in this manner, including a general description of the programs, the number of patients in treatment on the contact date, the number of staff dealing specifically with alcoholics, the availability of separate data on persons with alcohol-related problems, the administrative arrangements of the programs and, in short, all data that would indicate whether or not the agencies conformed to the survey definition of a treatment program. Many programs were found not to conform to the definition and were excluded from the survey. But it was also found that individual programs knew of other programs which were not on the master list; these were added and contacted, and many were found to conform to the survey definition.

Finally, after visiting every program on the master list, the mental health/mental retardation agencies of every county in the state were contacted in order to ascertain that the survey team had not missed any programs or that no new programs had developed since the original list was compiled. Several programs were thereby added to the list and visited. In this way, the comprehensiveness of the survey was maximized.

Collecting the Data

It was decided that in order to gain adequate information on the existing programs, it was necessary to conduct on-site visits. While it would have been less costly and time-consuming to collect the data by phone or mail, such procedures do not afford the opportunity to observe the programs as they actually operate in their own environment. In addition, the informal face-to-face interaction which was often so enlightening could never have developed over the phone or in a letter.

The site-visiting team was comprised of six members having a variety of backgrounds, including psychiatry, social work, sociology, anthropology, and public health. Teams of two or three visited each of the 84 programs, traveling over 30,000 miles in the process.* The site visiting was conducted over a 13-month period, from December 1972 to December 1973. It is pertinent to note that the sites were located and visited in two steps, beginning with the better known and easily identified programs throughout the state, followed by the more obscure and geographically isolated programs.

The interviews, which were conducted according to a questionnaire schedule, took between one and two hours. In most instances, the director of the program was interviewed, often accompanied by one or two staff members. The team was careful to emphasize that the questionnaire was not for the purpose of an evaluation but rather was simply a data collection instrument; the goal was to describe the state of the current treatment effort in the Commonwealth, not to pass judgment on it. This explanation of the purpose of the survey seemed to dispel some of the apprehension of program directors, and may have resulted in more sincere responses than might otherwise have been the case. Following the formal interview, the program directors usually conducted a complete tour of the facility.

By actually seeing the facility, the survey team was enabled to have a clear, concrete impression of the variety of physical settings in which treatment takes place in the Commonwealth. An independent rating of both the program's cooperativeness and the quality of treatment provided was made after leaving the site. The ratings were impressionistic in that no established treatment standards were used. They were made in an effort to discover not only what exists in terms of treatment facilities but also to provide a preliminary assessment of quality. As will be described in greater detail in a later chapter, these ratings were a meaningful first step toward evaluation of the treatment system.

After a short time, the team was convinced that site-visiting was by far the best way of collecting the information. There were both general and specific reasons for this conclusion. In general, there seemed to be no other way of arriving at a *gestalt* of the treatment scene in a given area. Specifically, the team had the rich experience of observing certain

* Out of 84 programs, 59 were visited by teams of two; 15 were visited by teams of three; and 10 by teams of four or more.

aspects of the treatment system which otherwise would have gone unnoticed, but which were crucial for an understanding of the treatment effort in Pennsylvania.

For example, plush, modern facilities were discovered within a few blocks of programs in condemned buildings without heat or proper ventilation. Programs located in the same community often had little or no knowledge of one another, often resulting in a duplication of effort.

In the case of a program located in a hospital, the site visitors inquired as to its exact location at the reception desk. The receptionist had never heard of the program even though, as it turned out, it was located only one floor below. This gave the researchers some indication of the general feeling, particularly in the medical profession, toward formal alcoholism treatment programs. This impression was confirmed in several other similar situations.

In still another case, the team visited a program which was located in a small town that was severely damaged by the floods in the summer of 1972. The director described in poignant detail the emotional destruction that was wrought by the flood and the heavy impact this had on his program.

Finally, in a more exotic vein, if it had not been for its mobility, the site visit team would have missed the opportunity of visiting the art gallery and youth centre of a millionairess, art collector, and former ecdysiast. Despite some local controversy surrounding her activities, she claimed to have helped dozens of young people who had abused drugs. While this "phenomenon" was not a part of the survey, it nevertheless provided some feeling for the town in which the alcohol program that was being visited was located.

In a more serious vein, the site visits also resulted in the discovery of several alcohol programs that were receiving public funds but were not functioning, on-going treatment enterprises in any sense of the word.[5] While this was not often the case, it occurred frequently enough to convince the survey team of the absolute necessity of on-site visits.

While the methodology described above certainly is not foolproof, and it is possible that some legitimate programs may have been missed, the survey team nevertheless was able to obtain sufficiently complete data in order to describe the current state of treatment in Pennsylvania. It is hoped this will provide a good start in the construction of a permanent treatment system for the care of alcoholics.

References

1. Adler, F., Moffett, A.D., Glaser, F.B., et al. *A systems approach to drug treatment.* Philadelphia: Dorrance & Company, Inc., 1974.

2. *Ibid.* p. 43.

3. *Ibid.*

4. Barrett, M. *The Pennsylvania state alcohol abuse and alcoholism plan for 1971-72.* Harrisburg: Commonwealth of Pennsylvania, Vol. *1:* A design for action, 1972, p. 30

5. Moffett, A.D., Greenberg, S.W., and Glaser, F.B. Non-programs in the management of drug and alcohol abuse. Presented at the National Drug Abuse Convention, Chicago, March 30-April 1, 1974. Published as Report Series No. 2, Governor's Council on Drug and Alcohol Abuse, Harrisburg, Pa., 1975.

Section Two

THE TREATMENT PROGRAMS

Chapter 3

Definition of Alcoholism and Goals of Treatment

To define is "to fix or mark the limits of; to determine the essential qualities."[1] In dealing with a problem, whether it be building a bridge, writing a song, curing cancer, or helping the alcoholic, one would assume that to have an understanding of the nature of the entity would be a prerequisite. How is one to write a song, if one has only a vague notion of what its components are, how to distinguish it from something that is not a song, and how to articulate its parts? By the same token, it would seem essential to have a clear-cut conception of the nature of alcoholism in order to attempt to alleviate the problem. But there is no general agreement on the nature of alcoholism. Neither researchers nor treatment professionals utilize anything even approaching a consensus definition. It is quite likely that this has contributed to the weaknesses in structure, cohesiveness, and direction that were found. If one is not certain of what the problem is, it will be difficult to find an answer.

The terms "alcoholic," "chronic alcoholic," "alcohol addict," and even "problem drinker" are bandied about, often with little attention to their implications. All of these words are used interchangeably in reference to an imperfectly conceptualized malady that is either a cause, an effect, or a correlate of excessive use of alcohol. On the other hand, several students of alcoholism (to use what is usually considered the most general term) have attached distinct meanings to each of these terms. As Roebuck and Kessler aptly state, perhaps it would be most accurate to think in terms of "alcoholisms" in order to infer a wide range of pathological behaviors—physical, psychological, and social—that are associated with alcohol abuse.[2]

In this chapter, we will explore the meanings of such words as alcoholism, alcohol addiction, and so forth. We will approach this problem initially from the perspective of the alcohol literature and then relate this to the Pennsylvania program directors' conceptualizations. Finally, the latter will be compared to the goals of treatment outlined by the directors, in order to delineate the relationship, if any, between the definition of the problem and the orientation toward its alleviation.

History of Terminology

The first expression attached to the pathological consumption of alcohol was "dipsomania." Introduced early in the 19th century by C. von Bruhl-Cramer, a German physician practising in Moscow, the term was first used to include all types of excessive drinking. In the mid-1800s it became associated only with periodic bouts of drunkenness, interspersed with periods of abstinence or even controlled social drinking. However, the term "dipsomania" fell into disuse in the 20th century and shows no signs of returning to general parlance.

"Chronic alcoholism" was first used in 1849 by Magnus Huss, a Swedish physician. It was applied to excessive drinking which produced a functional disorder in the nervous system. Here, the malady was linked with definite physiological changes. At the turn of the century the term was broadened to include "all the lasting disturbances of the psychic and physical functions produced by the habitual abuse of alcohol." Thus, this term was applied to the psychobiological *effects* of excessive consumption. More recently, the term has been used a number of ways, such as to designate a particular phase of alcoholism or simply to communicate its long-term quality.

At the turn of the century, the term "alcohol addiction" was introduced. It was applied to people who were believed to be unable to stop drinking even though it was causing them social, psychological, and physical damage. This emphasis on loss of control has remained a major theme in the definition of alcoholism for the last half dozen decades. As will be noted below, for some students of alcoholism, loss of control—as opposed to excessive drinking—is the sole criterion for determining addiction.[3]

The most recent addition to the alcohol abuse terminology is problem drinking. Here, the emphasis is on the functional impairments that are generally associated with the abuse of alcohol. Proponents of this perspective opine that physical, psychological, and social dysfunctions can be measured in relatively objective ways, while loss of control or inability to abstain are relative concepts. This being the case, they state that such terms as alcoholism and alcohol addiction should be dropped from usage in favor of the more operational term of problem drinking.

The terms above, with the exception of dipsomania and problem drinking, are used liberally throughout the literature to designate a rather vaguely conceived malady known as alcoholism. Unfortunately, they are used both as synonyms for alcoholism and as terms for specific types or phases of alcoholism, with little consensus as to the correct application. With this in mind, we will now explore the various meanings of the term "alcoholism."

Definitions of Alcoholism

In searching the literature for definitions, we could locate none which was precise but yet inclusive. Rather, each had a particular emphasis, such as the pattern of drinking, the psychological and biological changes caused by alcohol, or the social, psychological, and physical pathology produced by excessive drinking. Therefore, the definitions are categorized according to their particular emphasis.

Disease Concept. Perhaps the most publicized definition of alcoholism is that which emphasizes the physiological changes that are a direct product of excessive consumption of alcohol. It is stated that "... there is little question but that the history, symptoms, and signs of alcoholism form a recognizable pattern. In fact, there is little disagreement regarding the 'diseased' status of the subject addicted to a sedative drug, perhaps because of the measurable derangements of physiological function that usually accompany the use of the intoxicant...."[4] These changes, while purely physical, are observable on the behavioral level in that there is an inability to control either quantity or duration of intake, or both. Thus, alcoholism, according to this definition, is physiogenic, with unmistakable behavioral consequences.

More importantly, in its symptomatic presentation, prognosis, and treatment, it conforms to the accepted criteria of a disease. This orientation has been adopted by Alcoholics Anonymous and more recently by the American Medical Association and is the view most widely held by the public.[5,6] The conception that the alcoholic is sick rather than morally weak ("degenerate") has been largely responsible for the development and professionalization of services for alcoholism. It has resulted in a range of services being made available to the alcoholic that might not otherwise have obtained. However, this change in emphasis may have been more a function of public policy than a product of scientific progress in the understanding of alcoholism. The wide public acceptance of the definition is reflected by the fact that out of 80 alcohol programs in the Commonwealth, 24% define alcoholism as a medical disease (see Table 1).

Jellinek has been by far the most vocal proponent of the disease concept. While the physiological/behavioral nature of alcoholism has

TABLE 1

Definition of Alcoholism by 80 Programs

	No.	%
Medical disease	19	23.8
Part of psychiatric syndrome	14	17.5
Social problem	11	13.8
Religious sin	0	0.0
Medical disease plus social problem	4	5.0
Part of psychiatric syndrome plus social problem	2	2.5
Medical disease plus psychiatric syndrome plus social problem	20	25.0
Disease plus psychiatric syndrome plus religious sin	1	1.2
Medical disease plus psychiatric syndrome	3	3.7
Disease plus psychiatric plus social problem plus sin	4	5.0
Don't know	2	2.5
	80	100

been alluded to for over a century and a half, he is responsible for its current conceptualization. According to Jellinek's definition, there are two types of alcoholism, only one of which is properly called a disease.* In order to qualify as the disease type, known as alcohol addiction, five criteria must be met—increased tolerance to alcohol, adaptive cell metabolism, withdrawal symptoms, craving, and either loss of control or inability to abstain.[8] If these criteria are not met, the alcoholic is

* Actually Jellinek delineated not two but five distinct forms of alcoholism, which he called *alpha, beta, gamma, delta,* and *epsilon. Alpha* corresponds roughly to habitual symptomatic excessive drinking, a term which he used later in his writing. It refers to a psychological dependence on alcohol for the relief of physical or emotional pain. *Beta* alcoholism is confined mainly to the physical malfunctions that accompany excessive drinking; withdrawal, or true addiction is not included. Both *alpha* and *beta* may develop into actual alcohol addiction. *Epsilon* alcoholism is characterized by periodic bouts of drinking similar to what used to be known as dypsomania. Only *gamma* and *delta* are properly called addictive alcoholism in that excessive consumption has resulted in cell and tissue alteration. In *gamma* alcoholism there is a loss of control in that there is an inability to limit intake during drinking occasions but the individual does not need to drink constantly. It is found most commonly in the United States and northern European countries. *Delta* alcoholism is characterized by an inability to abstain for more than a day or two but amount of intake is controlled. This type is uncommon in the United States.[7]

labeled an habitual symptomatic excessive drinker. Here, there is no loss of control, and the basic problem is not alcohol but rather the array of social and psychological problems that result in excessive drinking. To be sure, this type of alcoholism represents a poor adaptation to personal problems, but the individual is still capable of controlling intake.[9] While both types of alcoholism can be regarded as a symptom of an underlying personality disorder, only in the disease type is there a loss of control, making alcohol *per se* the major problem.

As in most diseases, alcohol addiction represents a progressive deterioration, both physically and behaviorally. Jellinek delineated four phases of this progression, the pre-alcoholic symptomatic phase, the prodromal phase, the crucial phase, and the chronic phase. In each period, alcohol occupies an increasingly central portion of the individual's life. As the disease progresses, there are shorter periods of abstinence, less ability to control amount of intake, onset of physical symptoms, such as blackouts and finally delirium tremens, and an ever-increasing impact on the individual's personal life. Finally, in the chronic phase, his life is completely dominated by alcohol, and the emotional problems that may have precipitated the initial drinking have receded into the background.[10]

Impaired Social and Psychological Functioning. In direct contrast to the disease concept is the perspective that regards alcoholism as any form of excessive drinking which results in an impairment of social and psychological functioning. Here, the emphasis is not on physiological criteria, such as cell or tissue change, but rather on the importance that excessive drinking has on the individual's life. Whether or not there is a loss of control or inability to abstain is relatively unimportant. What matters is the social and emotional deterioration caused by drinking. As Clinebell states: "A person is an alcoholic if one or more of his major adjustments in living—health, vocational, social, or marital—is periodically or continually hampered by drinking."[11] Ten of the program directors (15%) defined alcoholism as a social problem and only two (2.5%) as a combination of psychological and social problems. It should be noted that when a respondent defined alcoholism as a social problem, there are two possible meanings. One interpretation is that alcoholism is a threat to the ongoing functioning of society. The other is that alcoholism is a threat to the social functioning of the individual, as in family and job situations. However, since the functioning of both levels is interrelated, the lack of precision is not problematic.

Compared to the disease concept, this approach is fairly recent. Several authors have adopted this perspective as the most pragmatic and realistic.[12,13] In fact, Cahalan recommends that the term alcoholism be dropped in favor of the more descriptive term, "problem drinking." He states that this expression focuses attention on the behavior rather than the individual, making the treatment of symptoms instead of causes the primary goal.[14] According to Plaut, another proponent of this position, "Problem drinking is a repetitive use of beverage alcohol causing physical, psychological, or social harm to the drinker or to others."[15]

Deviation from Cultural Norms. A third definition is based on the set of culturally-derived norms that determine the acceptable boundaries of social drinking. "Alcoholics are those whose frequent and repeated drinking of alcoholic beverages is in excess of the dietary and social usages of the community. . . ."[16] In this case, the emphasis is not on the physical and emotional pathology generally underlying excessive drinking or the social-psychological problems that are its accompaniment, but rather on a drinking pattern that exceeds the limits of acceptable behavior. This perspective is usually presented in combination with the social-psychological functioning perspective.[17,18] None of the respondents defined alcoholism in this way.

Labeling. The labeling perspective is derived from the normative definition of alcoholism. According to this: "Alcoholism is a label attached to a drinking pattern defined as deviant by the social control institutions."[19] Here, it is not the quantity or rate of consumption that defines an alcoholic but rather the reactions to this behavior by the official agents of social control, such as psychiatrists or the police. Even though two people may drink the same amount at the same frequency, one will be labeled an alcoholic, while the other will escape this stigma. The theory is that when the label of deviant is attached by an agent of society, the opportunities for behaving in a conventional manner are reduced, and the individual becomes even further entrenched in a deviant lifestyle. In the case of alcoholism, a whole range of variables contribute to this labeling process, such as frequency of drunkenness, violent behavior while drunk, visibility to labeling agents, and social context. While this is an intriguing orientation, it is not prominent in the literature, and it was not encountered anywhere in our survey of facilities.

Part of Psychiatric Syndrome. This conception of alcoholism does not focus on drinking *per se* but rather on the complex structure and functioning of the personality. Derived from the psychoanalytic perspective, this theory views alcoholism as a symptom of deep, underlying emotional conflict. Therefore, as with any other neurosis, psychotherapy by a specially trained person is required.[20] Fourteen (17.5%) of the program directors defined alcoholism as part of a psychiatric syndrome.

Moral Failing. According to the moral definition, alcoholism is a sign of a weak and downgraded spirit. Unlike most of the other perspectives, alcoholism is defined as a sin rather than an underlying physical, emotional, or social problem. In fact, drinking itself is considered a risky business at best, and alcoholism only its extension. Abstinence (not only for the alcoholic but for everyone) is essential, since drinking is the root cause of alcoholism. If one does not drink, then obviously one cannot become an alcoholic.

This orientation has always been a part of our culture. It reached its peak in terms of popularity and influence just prior to World War I and was the driving force behind the Temperance Movement, which eventually resulted in the passage of 1919 of the Volstead Act. Since the repeal of Prohibition, much of the moral fervor against alcoholism has declined, having been replaced in the public mind by the disease concept.[21,22] Significantly, out of 80 program directors interviewed, none defined alcoholism as a sin. Currently, its major proponents are the Rescue Missions and the Salvation Army (see Chapter 14).

It is apparent from the above that there is general disagreement as to the nature of alcoholism. If to define is to express the essential nature of an object in a clear and precise manner, it is evident that at the present time, we have no single generally agreed upon definition of alcoholism. This observation is reflected both by the diversity of responses and by the fact that over one-third (42%) of the respondents defined alcoholism in terms of two or more dimensions. While the majority of respondents viewed alcoholism as a one-dimensional phenomenon, a substantial minority perceived of it as having two, three, or four dimensions. However, the precise nature of the relationship between the dimensions was usually not expressed.

Of all the responses given, the most common (25%) was a combination of medical, social, and psychological factors. This incorporates the elements of most of the definitions found in the current alcohol literature—loss of control or addiction as a result of excessive consumption, expression of deep-seated emotional problems and the cause of further personality deterioration, and impairment of social functioning. However, it should be noted that combining unidimensional and multidimensional definitions, the disease concept emerges as the most prevalent: 64% of all definitions included this component, compared to 55% and 52% for psychiatric syndrome and social functioning, respectively. In addition, the moral component is markedly absent. Only five respondents (6%) included this dimension in their definition, and only in combination with two or more other aspects. Thus, the component variously known as morality, spirituality, sinfulness, and so on does not appear to be of major import in the conceptualizations that Pennsylvania treatment directors have of alcoholism. The unidimensional definitions discussed above in combination with the three-dimensional medical-psychological-social conceptualization account for most of the response variation.

Goals

It is a reasonable assumption that the definition of a problem will in some way influence the approach to its alleviation. Conceptualizations place limits around reality. The act of delineating the essential components of an object entails the inclusion of certain elements and the exclusion of others. When the object is defined as a problem, the elements included in the definition will, to some extent, determine the approach to the problem's solution. The extent to which this is the case largely depends on the precision of the definition—the more precise the definition, the more pre-determined will be the approach to the solution. It is important to point out that it is the *approach,* not the solution, that is at least partially determined by the definition. Solutions are worked out by such variables as individual effort and luck, entities essentially external to definitions. In any event, it is logically expected that the way in which a problem is conceptualized will serve to indicate certain approaches and eliminate others.

For this reason, we have decided to compare definitions of alcoholism to treatment goals. We would not expect anything even approaching perfect correspondence owing to the lack of precision in conceptualizing the problem. However, we supposed that there would be some variation in response and that some of this variation would be explained by the differences in definition. From an experimental perspective, we are interested in finding the degree of association between the independent variable of definition and the dependent variable of goals. For each definition, we have suggested the general implications for treatment that follow logically.

Disease Concept According to this definition, alcoholism is an addictive disease. Regardless of its etiology—inherited predisposition, emotional, or social—the excessive consumption of alcohol produces distinct organic changes. These changes are reflected in behavior in that there is a loss of control of quantity consumed or an inability to abstain for an indefinite period. It is this loss of control which is the root cause of the personality deterioration, defensiveness, marital difficulties, and employment problems that are often correlated with alcoholism. Therefore, the goal of treatment is to reverse, if possible, both the physiological damage caused by excessive drinking and the concomitant loss of control. Only in this way will it be possible to deal with related problems in social and psychological functioning. According to this position, abstinence, the permanent absence of alcohol from the system, should be the primary goal of treatment, and all alcoholics, regardless of their background, length of drinking, and so forth require this mode of treatment.

Impaired Social and Psychological Functioning In this case, the treatment goal is to help the alcoholic achieve an understanding of the interpersonal difficulties created by drinking and to provide him with the means to alleviate these problems. Often this is done through family and vocational counseling. Here, the essence of alcoholism according to the disease concept—loss of control—is not of primary relevance. Rather, any damage to social and psychological functioning caused by excessive drinking is sufficient to constitute alcoholism and must be dealt with as such. Thus, the emphasis is on helping the individual to become a productive member of the community. If abstinence is required to attain this goal, then it will be sought; if the individual is capable of drinking in a controlled, responsible manner, this is certainly permissable. Above all, it is an improvement in functioning that is desired.

Part of Psychiatric Syndrome Since this definition conceives of alcoholism as one symptom in an entire configuration of neurosis, the only viable treatment alternative is to discover the underlying conflicts which have produced this psychopathology. Therefore the goal of treatment would be to help the alcoholic gain insight into the weaknesses of his personality development. Once the neurosis is worked through, it follows that the symptom—excessive drinking—and other resulting personal problems will begin to recede.

Since these three definitions of alcoholism, either alone or in combination, account for most of the variation in response, only their implications for treatment will be used in the following analysis.

Frequency

Of the 80 programs, 27 (32%) mentioned a single goal. Abstinence was mentioned most often of the 27 responses, followed by social-psychological functioning, and psychiatric syndrome. Thus, abstinence is the single most frequent response, with respect to goals, as was the disease concept of alcoholism, with respect to the nature of the problem. However, these single responses account for only a relatively small proportion of the total number of responses.

The majority of responses (65%) involved two or more goals. Of these, three-quarters contained abstinence as one of the components.

TABLE 2

Goals of Treatment of 80 Programs

	No.	%
Abstinence	15	18.8
Work out emotional problems	2	1.2
Improve social functioning	10	12.5
Combination of abstinence plus emotional problems, social functioning, or both	36	46.2
Combination of emotional problems and social functioning, with or without increased periods of sobriety	15	18.8
Other	2	2.5
	80	100

As can be seen from Table 2, the combination of abstinence with social-psychological functioning was the most frequently encountered goal orientation, accounting for almost half of the total responses. Relatively few respondents (18%) did not include abstinence as a goal. For the programs espousing non-abstinence goals, a common strategy was to help the alcoholic in increasing his periods of sobriety rather than to insist on absolute abstinence; in a sense, these programs opted for relative instead of absolute sobriety. According to this position, complete abstinence is an unrealistic and self-defeating treatment objective. Preferably, treatment should be directed toward decreasing alcohol consumption, perhaps even training the alcoholic to drink in a socially accepted way. It is felt that this is a goal that the alcoholic can accept in that it does not create the pressures of having to give up alcohol forever. However, the respondents did not appear to espouse the view of behavior modification, in which abstinence is clearly not desired. According to this perspective, training the alcoholic to drink socially is a more appropriate treatment goal than abstinence, since moderate consumption is a socially acceptable, and even encouraged, mode of behavior in our society. In contrast, the program directors who did not mention abstinence as a goal implied that ideally this would be desirable, but given the personality characteristics and histories of many alcoholics, they felt that its complete achievement was not realistic.

At this point, it is appropriate to review briefly the debate on abstinence. Until recently, it was a forgone conclusion that abstinence was perhaps the single most important criterion in evaluating the success of treatment. This was based on the position that addictive consumption results in permanent physical and psychological changes, such that a single drink would immediately re-activate the loss of control syndrome. Further, according to this position, abstinence increases the likelihood that the individual will be able to make significant social and emotional improvements.[23] However, recent studies have indicated that some alcoholics may, in fact, be able to drink in a socially acceptable manner.[24-26] These studies, based on random samples of previously uncontrolled drinkers, report that between 4 and 10% of all treated alcoholics are able to drink socially. They suggest that in the course of treatment, as the patient is increasingly better able to cope with his problems, drinking will naturally come under control.[27] While abstinence may be achieved, and should at least be attempted, if the individual is unsuccessful he should not be considered a treatment failure. Interestingly enough, this position, which is most commonly associated with behavioral models of alcoholism,[28] may also be found in the work of those who view the problem from a psychodynamic perspective.[29]

Thus, the two goals of abstinence versus modified drinking represent distinctly different approaches to alcoholism. The abstinence goal represents the conception of alcoholism as a physiologically based disease. On the other hand, objectives that either do not take any stand on abstinence or seek mainly to increase the periods of sobriety imply a perception of alcoholism more in terms of psychological and/or social factors. Therefore, it is expected that a program director's definition of alcoholism should correlate at least to some extent with his treatment objectives.

Definition versus Goals

According to our reasoning, the cells on the diagonal of Table 3 should be the most heavily loaded. That this is not the case is an indication of a lack of correspondence, to some extent, between definitions and goals. As can be seen, most definitions of alcoholism have very little predictive power in terms of treatment objectives. For example, by knowing that a program director defined alcoholism as part of a psychiatric syndrome, one could not predict the most likely goals of his program. Only for two definitions, the disease concept and the combination of the disease concept with one or more other approaches, did the frequency distribution approximate our expectations. When alcoholism was defined solely in terms of the disease concept, 80% of the responses fell in the category of either abstinence or a combination of abstinence and one or more other goals. However, when it was defined in terms of both the disease concept plus other dimensions, only two-thirds of the responses were contained in the two corresponding goal categories. Thus, the predictive power of the disease combination definition does not appear to be as strong as that of the disease concept alone.

These findings have a number of implications. First it seems that the disease concept, or some variation of it, is pervasive in the treatment field. The same is true for its treatment implication, abstinence. In both cases, two-thirds of the responses are accounted for by a medically-oriented approach. This may be a reflection of the acceptance of the disease concept (along with the prognosis, "once an alcoholic, always an alcoholic") by the general public. Secondly, this conceptualization is by far the best predictor of goal response. The other definitions yielded responses that covered the full range of possible objectives. Furthermore, the predictive power of this orientation was increased when the disease concept was the sole definition given.

One possible explanation for this association is that the disease concept of alcoholism is the least vague of all the definitions. It gives strict criteria for the addiction to alcohol, including loss of tolerance, loss of control, and psychic craving. While these variables cannot be easily measured, they nevertheless provide a highly-structured framework upon which to base treatment. The major implication of this conceptualization is that abstinence is an absolute requirement. Regardless of other goals that may be considered important, abstinence is a direct implication of this definition. That such precision is not the

TABLE 3

Definitions of Alcoholism by 80 Programs by Goals

Definition / Goals	Disease		Psychiatric syndrome		Social problem		Disease combination		Non-disease combination		Don't know		Total
Abstinence	5	27%	3	22%	2	18%	4	13%	0	0%	1	50%	15
Work out problems	1	5%	0	0%	0	0%	0	0%	0	0%	1	50%	2
Improve functioning	1	5%	3	22%	2	18%	3	9%	1	50%	0	0%	10
Abstinence combination	10	53%	4	28%	4	36%	17	53%	1	50%	0	0%	36
Non-abstinence combination	1	5%	4	28%	3	28%	7	22%	0	0%	0	0%	15
Other	1	5%	0	0%	0	0%	1	3%	0	0%	0	0%	2
Total	19	100%	14	100%	11	100%	32	100%	2	100%	2	100%	80

case with other definitions is demonstrated by the data.

There is both an advantage and a disadvantage to the predictability of goals from definitions. The advantage is that a correspondence between the two variables is conducive to a tightly-structured program having a set of well-defined aims. It can be argued that a program with a clear-cut direction is more likely to have success than one in which the problem is only vaguely conceptualized and the goals loosely delineated. On the other hand, it can equally be argued that the association between definitions and objectives may lead to inflexibility. Since there is no single empirically verified definition of alcoholism as yet, perhaps it is more realistic to have a rather loose definition of the problem and a diversity of goals. In this way, the program is not locked into any one conceptual framework which may eventually be proven erroneous.

One final statement is in order. While the data indicate that at least for the disease concept there is some relationship between definition and goals, there remains little overall correspondence between the two variables. In fact, it appears likely that the interview raised issues that had heretofore been given little consideration by the programs. On a purely impressionistic level, the respondents were somewhat surprised at being asked to define the problem with which they were dealing and the goals to which their efforts were directed. This suggests that rather than being a reflection of the program's philosophical framework, the responses were produced to satisfy the interviewers. While surely this was not the case with all programs, the apparent lack of a firm theoretical background leading to well-delineated goals seemed to occur all too frequently.

References

1. Webster's Seventh New Collegiate Dictionary. Springfield, Mass.: G. & C. Merriam Co., 1971.
2. Roebuck, J.B. and Kessler, R.G. *The etiology of alcoholism: constitutional, psychological, and sociological approaches.* Springfield, Ill.: Charles C. Thomas, 1972.
3. Marconi, J.T. The concept of alcoholism. *Journal of Studies on Alcohol, 20:* 216-35, 1959.
4. Gitlow, S. Alcoholism: A disease. *In:* Bourne, P.G. and Fox, R. (eds.), *Alcoholism: progress in research and treatment.* New York: Academic Press, 1973, pp.1-9.
5. Haberman, P.W. and Sheinberg, J. Public attitudes toward alcoholism as an illness. *American Journal of Public Health, 59* (7): 1209-1216, 1969.
6. Mulford, H.A. and Miller, D.E. Measuring public acceptance of the alcoholic as a sick person. *Journal of Studies on Alcohol, 26:* 314-23, 1964.
7. Jellinek, E.M. *The disease concept of alcoholism.* New Haven: Hillhouse Press, 1960.
8. Jellinek, E.M. Phases of alcohol addiction. *Journal of Studies on Alcohol, 13:* 673-678, 1952.
9. Jellinek, E.M. Phases of alcoholism. *In:* Pittman, D.J. and Snyder, C.R. (eds.), *Society, culture, and drinking patterns.* New York: John Wiley & Sons, 1962, pp.356-368.
10. Jellinek. Phases of alcohol addiction. *op.cit.*
11. Clinebell, H.J. *Understanding and counseling the alcoholic.* New York: Abingdon Press, 1956, p.36.
12. Moore, R.A. The conception of alcoholism as a mental illness. *Journal of Studies on Alcohol,* 29: 172-175, 1968.
13. Mulford, H.A. Drinking and deviant drinking, U.S.A., 1963. *Journal of Studies on Alcohol,* 25: 635-650, 1964.
14. Cahalan, D. *Problem drinkers.* San Francisco: Jossey-Bass, 1970.
15. Plaut, T.F. *Alcohol problems: A report to the nation by the cooperative commission on the study of alcoholism.* New York: Oxford University Press, 1967, pp.37-38.
16. Clinard, M.B. *Sociology of deviant behavior,* 2nd Edition. New York: Holt, Rinehart & Winston, 1963, p.338.

17. Keller, M. and Efron, V. The prevalence of alcoholism. *Journal of Studies on Alcohol,* 20: 352-356, 1959.

18. Seeley, J.R. The W.H.O. definition of alcoholism. *Journal of Studies on Alcohol,* 20: 352-356, 1959.

19. Cahn, S. *The treatment of alcoholics.* New York: Oxford University Press, 1970, p.36.

20. Siegler, M., Osmond, H. and Newall, S. Models of alcoholism. *Journal of Studies on Alcohol,* 29: 571-591, 1968.

21. Haberman and Sheinberg. *op.cit.*

22. Mulford and Miller, *op.cit.*

23. Bolman, W.M. Abstinence versus permissiveness in the psychotherapy of alcoholism. *Archives of General Psychiatry, 12:* 456-463, May 1965.

24. Davis, D.L. Normal drinking in recovered alcoholics. *Journal of Studies on Alcohol,* 23: 94-104, 1962.

25. Gottheil, E., Alterman, A.I., Skoloda, T.E., et al. Alcoholic patterns of controlled drinking. *American Journal of Psychiatry, 130* (4): 418-422, April 1973.

26. Pattison, E.M., Headley, E.B., Gleser, G.C., et al. Abstinence and normal drinking: An assessment of changes in drinking patterns in alcoholics after treatment. *Journal of Studies on Alcohol, 23:* 610-633, 1968.

27. Bolman. *op.cit.*

28. Cahalan. *op.cit.*

29. Bolman. *op.cit.*

Chapter 4

A Practical Taxonomy of Treatment Programs

Introduction

One's use of past experience ought optimally to be flexible. While what has happened previously may be an invaluable guide, each new situation is unique and demands a creative approach. Simple and direct application from one situation to the next is therefore likely to be less than satisfactory. The experience of the survey team in devising a classification system for alcoholism treatment programs provides a gloss upon this text.

At the beginning of the survey, more by default than by conscious and deliberate decision, the taxonomy which had been developed for the drug abuse treatment program survey was incorporated in the instrument for the present survey. That system of classification[1] was based upon the nature of the principal means of intervention utilized by a given program. Thus, for example, some programs were classified as methadone maintenance programs if they chiefly relied upon the dispensing of that artificial narcotic for their therapeutic effect. Other programs, which utilized their own social structure as the principal therapeutic instrument, were classified as therapeutic community programs, and were further divided into three subtypes (residential, non-residential, and religious). In all, nine significantly different and mutually exclusive "modalities" of intervention were identified, and programs were all classified into one of them. The sole exception occurred in the case of a single program which made significant use of more than one intervention strategy.

In view of the considerable success of this type of analysis, it was carried over to the survey of alcoholism treatment programs with little modification (certain glaring discrepancies, such as the low probability of finding a methadone maintenance program for alcoholics, were naturally taken into account). From the very beginning, however, it seemed clear that the application of the drug program taxonomy to alcoholism programs was unworkable. A few programs, such as one therapeutic community program which treated both narcotic addicts and alcoholics, fell readily into the previous classification. But most programs proved more refractory to attempts at categorization. By the time the field work had been completed it had become abundantly evident that the classification embodied in the survey instrument was wholly unsatisfactory and would have to be abandoned. The fundamental reason was that most programs simply could not be distinguished from one another on the basis of the kind of intervention they offered.

For it was all the same. There was an essential monotony to therapeutic intervention in alcoholism programs that defied classification. This is, to be sure, an impressionistic conclusion, though it was forced upon the survey team by a practical problem—that of classifying programs. Direct data on intervention was not gathered as this was not a purpose of the survey as originally conceived. The discriminate characterization of therapeutic intervention is as yet an underdeveloped art, and it is questionable how it might be done even if approached intentionally. In this instance the team had to rely upon its experience with all programs, and its consensus was clear: treatment intervention in alcoholism programs was essentially the same from one program to the next, and hence could not form the basis for a taxonomic system.

Characterizing the therapeutic intervention which did occur is not an easy matter, and any such attempt will naturally do some violence to each of the 80 programs. But if there is yet some degree of variation, the team felt both that the degree of variation was small and that it occurred about a dominant mean. Thus, therapeutic intervention in the bulk of programs was low-key rather than intense. As a matter of fact, it was often casual. Generally speaking, it was not structured except to a modest degree; for example, neither the leadership of, nor membership in many group therapy sessions appeared to be constant. Leaders and members seemed to be viewed as more or less interchangeable, either between or within groups, and indeed their personal and career characteristics often seemed to be the same, irrespective even of whether an individual or group session was taking place. To say that the process appeared to be a modified version of the type of interaction usually seen at an Alcoholics Anonymous meeting, prudently detheologized and diluted so as to avoid any unfortunate implications which might accrue to the provision of no alternative, is surely limited and misleading, especially with respect to particular programs. But it was generally so. Pervading all was an attitude of mild pessimism, a feeling perhaps that the passage of time rather than formal intervention was the operative mechanism in eventual sobriety, and a realistic appreciation of the lack of formal training in more complex intervention techniques on the part of most persons responsible for intervention at the clinical level.

Further description is probably unwarranted. Those familiar with alcoholism treatment programs will (it is hoped) recognize what is being said, while those without practical exposure will need to acquire it before passing judgment upon the validity of the description. A further observation needs to be made: the team also felt that the monotony of intervention strategies was a secondary phenomenon. It seemed to be a result of the homogeneity of the population under treatment. Here were no stark, staring differences between individuals as had been observed in the drug treatment programs. Here were no startling dichotomies as between the white, middle class, hallucinogen-abusing "dope fiend" and the black, ghetto-dwelling, hard-core intravenous heroin addict. Here was a group of people who were very much the same. Their characteristics will be described in some detail in a later chapter. Impressionistically, they were a group of older white men of working-class origins and marginal general adjustment either accompanied by or due to chronic alcohol ingestion. They were familiar to their program, having been treated there many times before. They had few prospects and fewer illusions. They were depressed. They were entitled to be depressed.

There is no intention to imply that only such persons actually have problems related to alcohol. The team fully subscribed to the notion that alcoholism, whatever it is, is no respecter of persons. But it seemed clear that there had been a powerful labeling process (located in society rather than in the treatment programs) resulting in only a certain kind of individual obtaining access to designated alcoholism treatment programs in Pennsylvania. These programs were viewed as being exclusively for the chronic alcoholic, the chronic drunkenness offender, the individual far gone into an alcoholic lifestyle long before intervention was begun. What we were seeing was not so much the same type of individual as the combined, cumulative, and uniform effects of years of alcoholism, years of that peculiar kind of social processing which accompanies it, and the weight of other, concurrent social liabilities. Of course this is an unfair characterization of *all* persons in *all* programs; we readily admit that. But we also believe that the description is generally valid.

Thus the observation that intervention in the programs we visited was essentially monotonous is not *per se* a criticism. Given the

TABLE 1

Characteristics of the Components of Alcoholism Treatment Programs in Pennsylvania

Component	Function	Structure
I	Acute Intervention	Medical or non-medical
II	Evaluation	Centralized diagnostic centre
III	"Intensive" Intervention	Residential facility; day program
IV	Stabilization	Halfway house
V	Maintenance	Out-patient clinic; AA;
VI	Domiciliary Care	Some state Hospitals; rescue missions

seriously limited population being dealt with, their generally restricted prospects, the great general neglect of the problem, and the gross under-provision of funds and treatment facilities which has so long characterized this field of endeavor, those valiant individuals who have dedicated themselves to working under such adverse circumstances can hardly be castigated for an absence of variety. That alternative and specific intervention modalities exist elsewhere in the field of alcoholism intervention is not to be denied, either. But the responsibility for seeing that these techniques are implemented, and under less straitened circumstances, must become the responsibility primarily of those not immediately involved in the clinical situation. We can be only deeply appreciative of and grateful for the work they have done, the work that others would not do.

A Functional Taxonomy

Having suggested both that the population of individuals socially selected for treatment in alcoholism programs is quite uniform, and that the same is true of the treatment provided to them, it is time to leave these unfortunate facts to their further development in the final section of this book and to return to the practical dilemma of the survey team. Because they were unable to utilize a taxonomy of programs based upon the nature of intervention, they had to look elsewhere. After much discussion and thought, they found a viable alternative. The eventual scheme of classification was based upon the *function* of intervention rather than upon its nature. In other words, programs were classified on the basis of what they did, rather than how they did it. Six unitary functions were identified which, either alone or in combination, could characterize all of the 80 programs visited during the course of the survey. These functions included acute intervention, evaluation, intensive intervention, stabilization, maintenance, and domiciliary care. When existing treatment programs were viewed in the light of these functions, it became apparent that the separate functions were usually imbedded in characteristic programmatic structures having relatively specific configurations in time and space. Since it appeared that a comprehensive treatment system would necessarily subserve all of the six functions, it was decided to refer to the combination of a specific function with its characteristic structure as a *component*. This relationship is schematically outlined in Table 1.

Before describing these components in some detail it may be worth noting that they bear a logical relationship to each other. They posit not only a sequence of patient flow within a system of treatment but specific relationships to each other. In addition, they constitute a reasonably exhaustive analysis of the functional necessities for a comprehensive treatment system for this population of persons with problems related to alcohol (and possibly also for other kinds of service delivery systems). To facilitate a discussion of the individual components and their functional relationships, a simple diagram may be serviceable (Figure 1).

The Individual Components

I. *Acute Intervention.* It not infrequently happens that a person who is having problems related to alcohol will present initially as an acute physical, social, and/or psychological emergency. There must therefore be a major point of entry into the treatment system which is capable of dealing with all of these problems. In the past, far more attention was paid to the physical problems of patients, both from the standpoint of acute and chronic intoxication and of allied medical complications. As a result, the emergency room of a hospital or, less infrequently, a special hospital ward specifically set aside for the purpose, was the most common locus for such a component. More recently, under the influence of experience in Toronto, Canada and elsewhere[2] residential detoxification centres with a close relationship to hospitals but not physically a part of them have been developed. In addition to a staff well-trained to recognize medical complications of alcoholism, these facilities are well-equipped to deal with the social and psychological emergencies which often receive less attention in a purely medical environment. In practice, it has been found that only a small percentage of patients actually require hospitalization, though in the instances in which such attention is required it may be life-saving.

II. *Evaluation.* Once the acute situation has been dealt with, it is prudent to plan a future course of action in each case. The development of an individualized treatment strategy is also required for the occasional individual who does not present under emergency circumstances. In order for such planning to be meaningful, there must be a minimum of two intervention alternatives at this point; hence one would generally not expect to find an example of component II in a

Figure 1

Schematic Diagram of the Components of an Alcoholism Treatment System

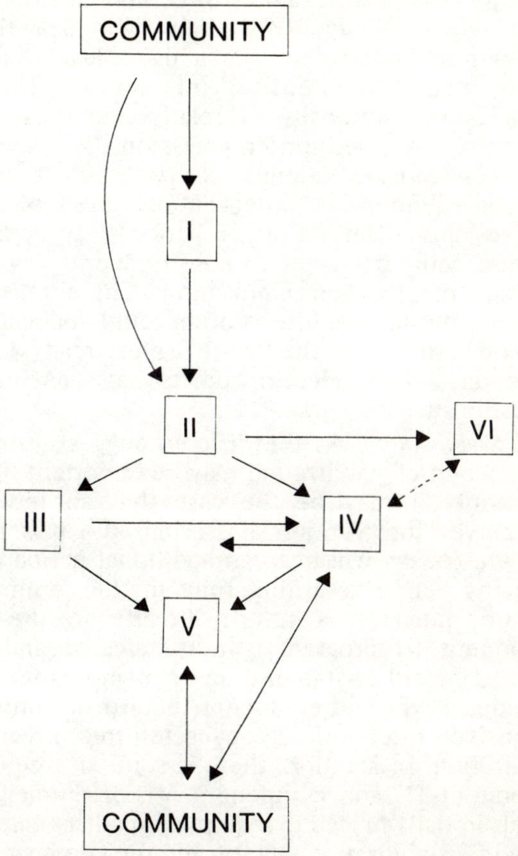

I — acute intervention
II — evaluation
III — "intensive" intervention
IV — stabilization
V — maintenance
VI — domiciliary care

treatment system with less than four elements (component I, component II, and two other components). Put another way, four-component programs may have a branched schematic design, while those having fewer components are linear. Practical considerations may lead to component I personnel performing component II functions, but such an arrangement would be less than ideal. The ability to deal with acute problems and the ability to make careful evaluations are different in themselves and require different support systems. In the drug treatment field, the "core" program[3] or the central medical intake is an example of component II.

III. *"Intensive" Intervention.* Should it appear that a given individual has potential for functioning at a higher level than currently, a decision may be made for "intensive" intervention. The reason for quotation marks is that intensity is relative, and (as was implied above) "intensive" intervention programs observed in the alcohol treatment field were not as intense as in the drug treatment field. Most commonly, "intensive" intervention takes place in both fields in a 24-hour residential setting over a period of approximately a month, that duration being determined more frequently by third-party insurance coverage than by clinical indications. There is no reason, however, why the locus of intensive intervention could not be a partial hospitalization program[4] even given the fact that more ready access to alcohol might create difficulties. Heroin addicts have been treated with relative success in such a program.[5]

IV. *Stabilization.* As the diagram suggests, components subserving the function of stabilization may be important for a variety of reasons. Commonly it may be the case that an individual who, through "intensive" intervention, has acquired a better level of functioning than previously, will need an additional period of time to consolidate his gains before returning fully to the community. Indeed, as the diagram indicates, a return directly to the community from a component III program is not indicated and ought ideally to be followed by either stabilization or maintenance. A certain number of individuals who either do not require or cannot take advantage of "intensive" intervention can be referred directly from evaluation to stabilization. In addition, there is some degree of resonance between component IV and component VI, or domiciliary care. Some individuals initially judged to require domiciliary care may prove capable of living in a stabilization facility, and the converse may also occasionally be true. A small arrow indicates that some people from component IV may return (or be sent for the first time) to component III for initial or additional "intensive" intervention. Thus its arrangements within the treatment system make component IV one of the most functionally versatile and hence one of the most critical components. This function is usually subserved by the halfway house, although variations such as the quarter-way house may also be found.

V. *Maintenance.* When individuals have achieved sufficient stability to return to virtual full-time life in the community, it may be desirable in most cases that they continue to receive some therapeutic input to maintain them at that level. Most commonly, these individuals will come either from component III or component IV. The system model suggests that, contrary to most current practice, an individual should under no circumstances be admitted directly to component V without a careful evaluation with respect to other alternatives. This reflects the fact that problems with alcohol tend to be chronic and severe, especially given the considerations relating to social selection for treatment noted above. Thus, out-patient treatment alone is unlikely to be productive of good results. The classic maintenance structure from a medical viewpoint has been the out-patient clinic. In the field of alcoholism the remarkable group, Alcoholics Anonymous, is responsible for a very large share of this component indeed (see Chapter 13).

VI. *Domiciliary Care.* Such are the effects of the chronic ingestion of alcohol and its complications that, over the long run, a certain number of individuals will be rendered permanently incapable of extramural community existence. These will often be persons with chronic organic brain damage. No one who has dealt with, for example, a person with Korsakoff's psychosis will see any merit in strenuous attempts to return most such patients to community life. It is unfortunate that these instances occur, but it is surely the better part of wisdom to recognize the fact. One such individual can place a truly astonishing burden upon the social resources of any community. In general, state hospitals have come to subserve the domiciliary function. However, in a very significant sense, missions also subserve this role (see Chapter 14).

The Functional Taxonomy Applied to Pennsylvania

It proved possible to classify the 80 Pennsylvania treatment programs visited during the survey by applying this functional taxonomic system. Naturally, a retrospective classification is far less satisfactory than one done *in statu nascendi* with the scheme firmly in mind. No doubt errors, both of omission and commission, have been made. Hopefully they will prove infrequent enough that the results may be considered valid. It should be kept in mind, of course, that time has necessarily elapsed between the completion of the field work on the survey and the appearance of this report. Hence the analysis is dated and reflects the past rather than the current scene.

The most fundamental finding of the survey was that some alcoholism treatment programs subserved only one function while others subserved more than one. That is, some programs had only one component while others had two or more. This is shown in Table 2, and was not unexpected. From a quantitative viewpoint, however, it is a matter for the most serious concern. More than 70% of all programs, at

TABLE 2

Alcoholism Treatment Programs in Pennsylvania
Having One or More Than One Component.

Components	No. Programs	% Programs	% Patients (N = 6805)
One	57	71.2	53.2
More than one	23	28.8	46.8
	80	100.0	100.0

TABLE 3

Alcoholism Treatment Programs in Pennsylvania
Having One or More Than One Component
By Geographic Area, in Percent

No. of Components	Metropolitan (N = 24)	Other (N = 56)
One	70.8	71.4
More than one	29.2	28.6
	100.0	100.0

TABLE 4

Alcoholism Treatment Programs in Pennsylvania
By Number of Components

No. of Components	No. Programs	% Programs	% Patients (N = 6805)
1	57	71.2	53.2
2	13	16.3	26.9
3	6	7.5	4.8
4	2	2.5	4.8
5	2	2.5	10.3
6	0	0.0	0.0
	80	100.0	100.0

the time of the survey, were single component programs, and these programs were serving more than half of all patients in treatment.

Such a situation may be in the grand tradition of entrepreneurial treatment, but it is a horror show from a systems viewpoint. With certain notable exceptions, such as Allegheny County, it was clear to the survey team that most single-component programs operated in splendid isolation. If they related at all to components subserving functions different from their own, the relationship was highly informal and subject to great variation. Any system burdened with a large proportion of unrelated single component programs is highly unlikely to render comprehensive care.

To dispose quickly of one argument which might be advanced to rationalize this state of affairs: it could be argued that only large cities would have the resources required to support multi-component programs. However, a geographic breakdown reveals a virtually exact split; just over 70% of the programs in both metropolitan and in other areas are single component programs (Table 3). It seems, therefore, that the preponderance of single component programs is not a function of population density, availability of resources, availability of personnel, or other distinguishing characteristics of large cities. Rather, it seems that there may have been a general lack of conceptualization of the treatment of alcohol-related problems in systematic terms.

Nor can much comfort be taken in the fact that only slightly less than half of the patients in treatment were being seen in programs having more than one component. Table 4 provides a further breakdown of treatment programs by the number of components which they contain. It may be seen that there is an inverse relationship between the number of components and the number of programs. Another way of expressing this is that the more comprehensive a program is, the less likely it is to be found in Pennsylvania. More than half of the patients who were being treated in programs with more than *one* component were being treated in *two* component programs—something of an improvement, but not impressive. As noted above, a four-element program is required in order to make a realistic component II a functional part of the treatment system; that is, it is only in programs with four or more elements that a reasoned decision concerning the optimum course of treatment is likely to be made. Almost 85% of all patients were *not* receiving treatment in such programs.

Moreover, *no* programs were found which contained all six of the elements posited by the theoretical model as being necessary for a comprehensive system. One could perhaps argue that, while individual *programs* might not possess all six elements, there might be several programs within a community which, taken together, might provide all six elements, and hence the community might be said to have a comprehensive program. Certainly there is some validity to such a claim and, in the presence of a large number of individual component programs, assuring that such a mix did indeed occur might be a worthwhile objective. In practice, this does not happen frequently. The survey team found only one community in Pennsylvania which had effective access to all six components. Moreover, the existence of all six components does not necessarily imply that they relate functionally and smoothly to each other in a systematic manner.

Moving now to a consideration of the degree to which each of the separate components was utilized within the Commonwealth, it is possible to view the data in two ways. One is to look only at the single component programs; the other is to look at the utilization of a given component *in toto,* whether it is a free-standing program by itself or a part of a multi-component program. Both sets of data appear in Table 5, the first column enumerating the 57 single component programs and the second the 119 separate components of all 80 programs. One glaring fact emerges: considered either way, the treatment system at the time of the study was dominated by a single component (V). Over 60% of single component programs consisted of these out-patient clinics, and almost half of all components were of this kind. This seems a particularly important and unfortunate occurrence. It implies a lack of vigor in the overall treatment approach, a tendency to accept an impaired level of functioning and to make, perhaps at best, a half-hearted effort to maintain even that. Such a level of effort may be realistic for a small number of patients, but even then it ought to be provided as a matter of reasoned choice and not necessitated by default. While the out-patient clinic has an important role to play as a part of an overall treatment system, perhaps even a crucial role, it is hardly satisfactory as the backbone of an entire state effort. Yet at the time of

TABLE 5

Utilization of Individual Components in Pennsylvania Treatment Programs, Percent

Component	In Single Component Programs (N = 57)	In All Programs (N = 119)
I	3.5	15.1
II	0.0	3.4
III	15.8	19.3
IV	17.5	14.3
V	61.4	44.5
VI	1.8	3.4
	100.0	100.0

TABLE 6

Utilization of Treatment Components Alone or in Combination with Other Components

Component	Use Alone	Use in Combination
I	2	16
II	0	4
III	9	14
IV	10	7
V	35	18
VI	1	3
	57	62

the survey, this was the position it occupied by the sheer weight of its prevalence.

It is also of some interest to consider the degree to which the separate components are utilized alone, as single component programs, as compared with their use in combination with other components. Table 6 indicates that, of the six components, two (IV and V, or out-patient clinics and halfway houses) are more frequently used alone, while the four other elements are usually found in combination. In both instances this reflects principally the logic inherent in the programs themselves. Out-patient clinics and halfway houses easily stand on their own and maintain their viability in a competitive and unplanned system. And while on the surface it appears consonant with a systems perspective that four of the six components are more commonly found in combinations, closer investigation dispels this view. Only 5% of all programs have four or more components. Most multi-component programs are of the "short-chain," linear variety, with 19 of 23 or 83% containing only two or three components (see Table 4). No independent evaluation programs exist to link single-component programs together rationally (see Table 5). It seems to be a logistical need for feeder and follower programs in order to accomplish such mundane ends as the maintenance of a high census which accounts for the many "short-chain," linear combinations, more than the desire to provide a comprehensive approach to treatment with a branched schematic design.

Finally, it is interesting to ask what the pattern of components would look like under ideal circumstances, and how this compares with matters as they were found. One way of constructing a treatment system would make this comparison difficult, since with close functional interrelationships between single, dual, or triple component programs some functions could be consolidated and, for example, one domiciliary could serve several small systems of components. But this has not been the pattern up until now. Where comprehensive care has occurred, it has been in terms of uniting all components of care under one administrative (if not physical) roof. Assuming that this pattern were to continue, the theoretical model (Figure 1) would predict one of each kind of component for each such system. Since at the time of the survey there were 119 components in existence, they may be compared with a hypothetical 120-component system containing 20 of each of the six components (Table 7).

When this is done the imbalances of the present system are readily visible. As was suggested by the raw figures the dominant feature is a gross over-supply of component V, out-patient clinics subserving the function of maintenance. In terms of under-supply, there would appear to be a palpable need for both evaluation and domiciliary programs. Other components are more or less represented as they would be under ideal circumstances. It is nevertheless instructive that both acute intervention and stabilization facilities are under-represented as compared with the ideal; this corresponds with the recommendations of program directors in Chapter 9 that more detoxification and halfway facilities are needed. Apparently the need for evaluation and domiciliary facilities is not obvious except from a systems perspective. Their failure to appear in recommendations confirms the preoccupation of program personnel with pressing present needs.

Summary

The survey team found that it was unable to apply to alcoholism programs the descriptive taxonomy which had been utilized for drug treatment programs. The latter had been based upon the nature of the therapeutic intervention. Intervention seemed to be thoroughly uniform in the alcoholism field, possibly reflecting the uniformity of

TABLE 7

Existing Components of Pennsylvania Alcoholism Treatment Programs Compared with Ideal as Predicted by Theoretical Model (Fig. 1)

Component	Existing	Ideal	Difference
I	18	20	− 2
II	4	20	−16
III	23	20	+ 3
IV	17	20	− 3
V	53	20	+33
VI	4	20	−16
	119	120	

the patient population being generated for the programs by the social process of labeling. Therefore a revised taxonomy based upon the function rather than the nature of intervention was devised and applied retrospectively (with all the hazards attendant upon such a strategy) to the 80 programs. Six functional components were identified which, alone or in combination, were capable of characterizing all of the treatment facilities. These components could be related to each other in a logical and dynamic manner in the context of a model comprehensive treatment system design.

Application of this scheme of analysis indicated that more than 70% of existing programs were single component programs, and that more than half of all patients were being served in these programs. They were the dominant type of program both in the metropolitan districts of the state and elsewhere. Indeed, there was an inverse relationship between comprehensiveness and availability of programs: the more components a program contained, the less likely it was to exist, and no program was found which contained all six components. Eighty-five percent of all patients in treatment were in programs containing fewer than four components, a configuration minimally necessary to offer meaningful treatment alternatives.

The treatment system at the time of the survey was dominated by component V programs subserving the function of maintenance, principally out-patient clinics. These constituted more than 60% of the single component programs and almost half of all existing components. Most frequently found existing on their own rather than in combination with other programs, they were in great over-abundance when compared with the theoretically-predicted need for them. This seemed to reflect the ease with which such a facility may be established and the general absence of a determined approach to the treatment of alcoholism.

In the final analysis, all of these facts add up to a most unfortunate lack of planning and organization of treatment. While this needs to be pointed out repeatedly as it is supported by the data, there is no intention of imputing blame. The treatment enterprise in general has not, to date, included a systems perspective in its repertoire. Rather, treatment has been a bastion of rugged individualism, and has attracted individuals having both the desire and the ability to function on their own. Such an orientation is not necessarily antithetical to an organized and structured systems-oriented approach, and in many instances they complement each other. A rational system can provide a therapist with a much more solid base of operations. But until a systems perspective is included in the *training* of therapeutic personnel, they may not recognize this fact. Although the asystematic aspects of treatment cry out for fairly immediate action, the inclusion of a systems perspective in therapeutic training programs may help to prevent such clinical chaos in the future.

References

1. Adler, F., Moffett, A.D., Glaser, F.B., et al. A systems *approach to drug treatment.* Philadelphia: Dorrance & Co., 1974.

2. O'Briant, R.G. and Lennard, H.L. *Recovery from alcoholism: A social treatment model.* Springfield: Charles C. Thomas, 1973.

3. Glaser, F.B. The treatment of drug abuse in the rural South: Application of the core-shell treatment system model. *Southern Medical Journal,* 67: 580-86, May 1974.

4. Glaser, F.B. The uses of the day program. *In:* Barten, H.H. and Bellak, L. (eds.) *Progress in Community Mental Health, vol.2,* New York: Grune & Stratton, 1972, pp.221-48.

5. Kaufman, E. A psychiatrist views an addict self-help program. *American Journal of Psychiatry. 128:* 846-52, January 1972.

Chapter 5

The Patient Population

Chapter 5

The Patient Population

In order to gain insight into the magnitude of any social problem, it is necessary to have valid and reliable estimates of both the prevalence of the problem in a given population at a particular period of time and the type and extent of social intervention for this problem. Only by comparing these two sets of data can a treatment system make informed policy decisions concerning the specific needs of the population at hand. One of the central concerns of this survey is to provide a description of the characteristics of alcoholics in treatmnet in Pennsylvania. However, where there are available data, we would also like to provide comparisons on a very gross level between the treatment population and the general population of alcoholics. In this way, not only can we learn the characteristics of those already in treatment but also the characteristics of those who may not have entered treatment.

Estimating the Prevalence of Alcoholism

Since the 19th century, a number of procedures has been developed for estimating the prevalence of alcoholism in a given population. Some of these have depended upon such indicators as officially recorded deaths from alcoholism, drunkenness arrests, hospital admissions for alcoholism, alcohol consumption rates, surveys of drinking practices in the general population, and deaths from cirrhosis of the liver.[1,2] Of all of these, estimates based upon cirrhosis deaths are perhaps the best known and most widely used.

In the early 1940s, Jellinek developed a formula for the indirect estimation of alcoholism in a general population by using the total number of deaths annually from liver cirrhosis.[3] This formula assumes a constant relationship between cirrhosis deaths and alcoholism with complications.[4,5] Based on this formula, Jellinek estimated that one out of every 15 adults who use alcohol is an alcoholic.[6] Jellinek's work has undergone considerable criticism, generally for under-representing the prevalence of alcoholism.[7,8] However, studies using independent, and in some instances more direct, methods of estimation have yielded results so similar to Jellinek's that it is probably safe to assume that it is a reasonably accurate measure.[9-11] In addition, several other studies have substantiated the close correlation between alcohol consumption and cirrhosis, both on the individual and aggregate levels.[12-15] Therefore, estimates based on cirrhosis mortality rates are probably adequate in terms of planning a treatment system, even though alternate methods, such as direct estimates based on survey samples of alcohol consumption, have some advantages and should be further developed.

Prevalence of Alcoholism in the United States

Virtually all studies, using various methods of estimation (cirrhosis mortality, alcohol consumption, direct survey), report a sharp increase in the prevalence of alcoholism between the end of World War II and the present. While various definitions of alcoholism have been used, it is generally agreed, based on national samples, that between 4 and 9% of all adults are classified as excessive drinkers whose drinking has impaired their social, psychological, and physical functioning.[16-19] Whether this group should be called alcoholics, problem drinkers, or simply excessive drinkers is a moot point with respect to intervention; it represents a population that is probably in need of treatment. The discrepancies in the various estimates are the result of differences in both procedure and definition. Jellinek's estimate, which is at the low end of the range, was derived from his formula using the cirrhosis death rate. The other three were based on interviews of randomly selected national samples. Two studies fell in the middle of the range of estimates. Cahalan et al (1969) defined what was referred to as "heavy escape drinking" in terms of a combination of frequency-quantity and expressed reasons for drinking. Mulford's estimate was based on a combination of frequency-quantity and social functioning. At the high extreme of the range was the Cahalan (1970) study, in which problem drinking was defined in terms of an 11-point scale of physical, psychological, and social functioning.

In terms of demographic characteristics, there is also a remarkable degree of consensus in the literature. The prevalence of problematic excessive drinking has universally been found to be greater among males than among females, often to the order of magnitude of three, four, or more.[20-24] The proportion of blacks with drinking problems is usually found to be greater than the proportion of whites. However, this difference is largely explained by the over-representation of black females among alcoholics. Most studies show that black males have the greatest proportion of problem drinking, white males and black females are approximately equal, and white females have by far the lowest prevalence.[25-28] It has been suggested that in our society, the drinking habits of black females are similar to those of males in that their social role has traditionally been one that is associated with maleness.[29] Owing to the historical discrimination against black males in the job market, black females have been forced to take on financial and decision-making responsibilities in the family. Thus, it is hypothesized that since black females "act" like males in the social sense, the collective sentiments proscribing excessive (and public) drinking among females are somewhat loosened.

The age range within which excessive drinking is concentrated has been found to be between the early 20s and the late 50s. After the age of 60, the prevalence of alcoholism drops off sharply.[30-36] However, there is a significant difference by sex in that the onset of excessive drinking among females occurs at a much later age, generally the early 30s.

There is a further consensus in terms of the correlation between population density and prevalence of alcoholism. In several national samples of the non-institutionalized adult population, it was found that excessive drinking—and drinking in general—is more prevalent in urban areas.[37-39]

The final major social characteristic is socioeconomic status, usually measured by education and occupation. Here, the evidence is more contradictory than is the case for sex, race, age, and population size. Some studies have found a strong inverse relationship between social class and excessive drinking,[40-42] while others find the greatest concentrations in both the lowest and highest levels.[43] It is possible that those studies finding an inverse correlation merely reflect the spiral of downward mobility experienced by many alcoholics; in other words, a confusion of cause with effect. However, an equally plausible explanation posits the existence of a lower-class subculture in which excessive drinking is a common reaction to personal problems.

Prevalence of Alcoholism in Pennsylvania

As of 1953, Pennsylvania ranked 14th in the nation in the rate of alcoholism.[44] In the last two decades, its rank has ascended only slightly; in 1970 it was 12th in rate of alcoholism and fourth in absolute numbers of alcoholics.[45] However, that alcoholism is a serious and growing problem in this state is beyond question. While there was only a 5% increase in population between 1962 and 1972, deaths from alcoholism and liver cirrhosis increased by 86% and 33%, respectively, in the same period.[46] (Some of this increase may be a function of improved diagnosis and greater frankness on the part of physicians in reporting the cause of death, but it is beyond doubt that a substantial portion of the increase is actual.)

In order to gain some insight into the numbers of Pennsylvanians in need of treatment for alcoholism versus the number actually receiving it, we compared the demographic data collected in a survey of drinking practices in the general adult population of this state with the demographic characteristics of the treatment population.

According to the study of Schaps and Rubin, over 631,500 people consume four or more drinks per day, which represents 7.3% of the entire adult population.[47] Similar to other studies of this type, respondents who reported this level of daily consumption were defined as "very heavy users" rather than alcoholics. It is a safe assumption that such people are in need of treatment, regardless of the labels attached. We will regard this as a valid estimate since it is in close agreement with the estimates reported above based on national samples.* In the present survey, a total of 6,805 alcoholics were receiving treatment at the time of the initial data collection. This represents only 1% of the total number in probable need of treatment. However, to assume that the remaining 99% are not undergoing treatment of any kind would be grossly inaccurate. Many treatment sources were not included in the present survey, such as private psychiatrists, mental health clinics without separate alcohol programs, industrial programs, and Alcoholics Anonymous. Nevertheless, we feel quite certain that vast numbers of alcoholics in the Commonwealth are receiving no treatment of any kind. At the very least, we may state that only 1% are being treated by programs that are recognized by some official agency as being facilities for the treatment of alcoholism. (See Chapter 2.)

Sex. According to the Schaps and Rubin study, 12.8% of the males in their sample consumed four or more drinks a day, compared with 2.8% of the females. Converting these proportions into numbers of excessive drinkers in the Commonwealth by sex, we estimate that there are approximately 517,400 males and 127,600 females in need of treatment for alcoholism.** We found a total of 5,505 males and 1,300 females in treatment in the facilities surveyed. In each case,

* This estimate is considered to be conservative. The Brenner formula, which utilizes cirrhosis deaths, has estimated the prevalence of alcoholism in Pennsylvania at 944,000.[60]

** This does not add up to 631,500, owing to the slight under-representation of males in the Schaps-Rubin sample. The same is true for race, in which whites are under-represented in the sample.

approximately 1% of the total population of alcoholics is being treated in the facilities included in the present study. Thus, each sex is proportionately under-represented in treatment according to the prevalence of the problem in the general population.

However, there is some reason to suppose that neither surveys of drinking practices nor of treatment facilities reflects the actual number of females who drink excessively. In contrast to the present study, others have found a marked under-representation of females in treatment for alcoholism.[48,49] In our society there are definite norms against drinking among women, particularly in public. Therefore, it is suggested that not only do women tend not to seek treatment for a drinking problem, but they may also be hesitant to admit to excessive drinking on a questionnaire. Since our figures on the representation of females in treatment are derived from questionnaire data, it is likely that there are a large number of alcoholic women who never come to the attention of either survey researchers or treatment personnel. Although there is no conclusive evidence, it is possible that women are in fact under-represented in treatment. As Lisansky states, " . . . they are, for the most part, a group which keeps out of public view and out of difficulty in the community."[50] For women in particular, alcoholism seems to be very much a hidden addiction. Thus, if we are to have a comprehensive treatment system, we may need to get a greater proportion of women out of the living room and into treatment.

Race The Schaps and Rubin study found that 10.9% of the non-white sample and 6.5% of the white sample consumed four or more drinks per day. Extrapolating these proportions to the total adult population, we estimate that there are approximately 513,200 whites and 74,000 non-whites in need of treatment. We found a total of 4,853 whites and 1,952 non-whites in treatment at the time of data collection. Whites appear to be somewhat under-represented in the treatment system, since only .08% of the total estimated population of white alcoholics are being treated, while for non-whites the proportion is approximately 2.5%. However, it must be kept in mind that the present survey did not include such treatment sources as private psychiatrists, industrial programs, and AA, in which whites, particularly of upper-middle and upper-socioeconomic status are often disproportionately represented. In contrasts, blacks may be more likely to be referred by various social agencies to publicly funded programs for the treatment of alcoholism.

Combining both race and sex, we find the patient population statistics to be dominated by black males. While this group comprises 4.2% of the total population in this state, they represent one quarter (24.3%) of the alcoholics in treatment. In general, males dominate the system, with females, particularly white females, accounting for a very small portion compared to their numbers in the population. (See Table I.)

Non-white females in treatment were represented in exact propor-

TABLE 1

Race—Sex Characteristics of Alcoholics in Treatment As Compared to the General Population of Pennsylvania

	Treatment		Pa. Population (1970)	
	No.	%	No.	%
Males	5,505	80.8	5,665,414	48.0
Females	1,300	19.1	6,138,910	52.0
Whites	4,853	71.3	10,737,732	91.0
Non-whites	1,952	28.6	1,066,592	9.0
White males	3,850	56.5	5,169,496	43.8
Non-white males	1,655	24.3	495,918	4.2
White females	1,004	14.8	5,568,236	47.2
Non-white females	296	4.3	570,624	4.8
Total	6805		11,804,324	

tion to their actual total numbers. While there are many plausible explanations to account for this finding, one reason may be that black female alcoholics are more visible than white females. As suggested above, within the black community the norms against women drinking in public may not be as strong as in other communities. Thus, it is suggested that alcoholism among black females would not be as well hidden as it may be among white females, and would thereby be more likely to come to the attention of such official social agents as social workers and police.

Age. According to studies of the prevalence of alcoholism, the great majority are in the 20-59 age group. Alcoholics in treatment in Pennsylvania are heavily weighted toward the older end of the range. Each respondent was asked the average age and the age range of alcoholics in treatment. For all programs, the average age was 42 with a range from 22 to 66 years of age. A substantial body of data indicates that while the great majority of alcoholics are in the 20-59 range, a wide range of serious social, psychological, and physical problems that are closely associated with excessive drinking are most likely to manifest themselves in the 20s and early 30s. Cahalan found that males in their 20s were more likely than any other age group to show dysfunctions, such as job and marital problems, alcohol-induced belligerence, frequent intoxication, and binge drinking.[51] Another study found that physiological dysfunctions associated with escessive alcohol consumption, such as black-outs, convulsions, and tremors, tend to manifest themselves in the middle 30s.[52] Still another study indicated that in Pennsylvania, as of 1960, cirrhosis of the liver contributed more to the risk of death from all causes in the 25-29 age group than in any other age.[53]

TABLE 2

Average Educational Level of Patients in Treatment

Average Education	No.	%
College graduate	2	2.5
College attendance	3	3.8
High school graduate	31	38.7
High school attendance	38	47.5
9th grade or lower	5	6.3
No response	1	1.2
Total	80	100.0

TABLE 3

Average Occupational Status of Patients in Treatment

Average Occupation	No.	%
Professional	0	0.0
Upper level executive	2	2.5
White collar	2	2.5
Blue collar—skilled	43	53.4
Blue collar—unskilled	19	24.2
Unemployed (nonskilled)	13	16.2
Derelict—skid row	0	0.0
No response	1	1.2
Total	80	100.0

Therefore, our finding suggests that the typical alcoholic either does not seek help or is not socially defined as being in need of help until his physical, personality, and social deterioration are in an advanced stage. This gap between the onset of deterioration and therapeutic intervention may be as long as 20 years.

Socioeconomic Status. When asked about the average educational level of their patients, three-quarters of the program directors reported that on the average their patients had either attended high school or graduated from it. With respect to employment, the positions held by most patients were characterized as either blue-collar skilled or unskilled. (See Tables 2 and 3.)

There are several plausible interpretations of these data. One is that they support the findings of studies that indicate that the prevalence of alcoholism is inversely related to social class position. A second explanation is that since alcoholism often leads to impairment of social functioning, there is substantial downward mobility. Hence, low

TABLE 4

Number of Alcohol Programs and Alcohol Patients in Treatment, by County Type[1]

County Type	1970 County Pop.		Programs		Alcoholics in Treatment	
	No.	%	No.	%	No.	%
Urban	3,553,625	30.1	24	30.0	3,127	46.0
Suburban	1,223,834	10.3	9	11.3	742	10.9
Small City	3,889,873	32.8	24	30.0	1,582	23.2
Rural	3,136,992	26.8	23	28.7	1,354	19.9
Total	11,804,324	100.0	80	100.0	6,805	100.0

[1] This is a summary table. The complete table can be found in Appendix A-1.

occupational status is an effect rather than a contributing factor. (This explanation, however, cannot account for the low educational level found in our survey.) Thirdly, there is a widely held hypothesis that class position determines the type of treatment. According to this explanation, which has been researched in the context of both mental illness in general and alcoholism in particular, upper-class people are most likely to be treated in intensive psycho-therapy by a psychiatrist in a private practice or hospital. At the other extreme, lower class people tend to be treated by organic therapy or custodial services in state or veterans' hospitals with comparatively less attention from highly-trained professionals.[54-59]

Owing to the extreme skewness of the present data for the two variables of class and treatment, it would be impossible to test this last hypothesis. However, we did find that the modal occupational group, skilled blue-collar, was also concentrated in the most frequent type of treatment, long-term maintenance, usually on an out-patient basis. Slightly more than half (53.5%) of the 43 programs which reported skilled blue-collar workers as the average occupational status of their patients were of the out-patient maintenance treatment type. This was also the case with the next most prevalent group, unskilled blue-collar workers (44.9% of 19 programs). Thus, while the class-treatment hypothesis cannot be tested in the present study, the results are quite consistent with it. Pennsylvania treatment programs, as we have defined them, are dominated by middle and working class alcoholics receiving treatment at community out-patient clinics.

With respect to the current educational and occupational activities of the individuals in treatment, we found that only 4.1% were involved full-time in an educational curriculum (3.2%, 0.6%, and 0.3% in vocational school, college, and public school, respectively). An approximately equal number of patients were either employed full-time (44.4%) or receiving public assistance (41.6%). As would be expected, a higher proportion of males than females were employed—46.0% of the males versus 37.5% of the females. Assuming the categories of full-time employment and public assistance are mutually exclusive, 14% are receiving other means of financial support, most probably from family members.

Population Size: Distribution of Programs and Patients According to the Schaps and Rubin study, excessive alcohol consumption is concentrated in the urban areas of Pennsylvania, specifically Philadelphia and Pittsburgh; excessive drinking was least common in the rural countries of the state. For purposes of comparison, the organization of the present data was patterned after this study. The programs were grouped into four categories, according to the population size of the county in which they were located. (see Tables 4 and 5. These are summary tables; the complete tables are found in Appendices A-1 and A-2. Category I represents urban counties; Category II, suburban counties; Category III, counties dominated by towns and small cities, and IV, rural counties.)

In order to estimate the extent to which need is met by intervention, comparisons are made between the geographical distributions of four elements—programs, patients, prevalence of alcoholism, and population. We are interested in determining the proportionality of patients and programs, patients and prevalence of alcoholism, programs and prevalence, programs and population, and patients and population.

We found that the distribution of *programs* by counties very closely approximated the distribution of the general population. The two exceptions were Philadelphia and Allegheny counties. Allegheny County, with 13.6% of the population, had 21.2% of the programs; Philadelphia County with 16.5% of the population, had 8.8% of the programs. However, in general, the distributions of programs and population were proportional.

In terms of *patients* in treatment, programs in urban counties were seeing a disproportionately large share of the patients in treatment; indeed, nearly half of all patients were in urban programs. Conversely, programs in small city and rural counties had a smaller proportion of patients in treatment than could be expected from their numbers in the population. However, when the distribution of patients is compared with the distribution of need, a rather surprising picture emerges (see Table 5). Areas comprised predominantly of small cities appear to be substantially under-represented with respect to patients. For every 149 alcoholics in such areas, there is only one in treatment as compared to a ratio of 139:1 for the entire state. It can be seen that areas dominated by small cities have the highest alcoholic-to-patient ratio in the state. From this finding it can be hypothesized that on the one hand, small cities are sufficiently similar to large cities in terms of such elements as density, heterogeneity, and transience which are often thought to

TABLE 5

Prevalence of Alcoholism and Prevalence of Treatment by County Type[1]

County Type	1970 pop.	Estimated Alcoholics[2]	Rate of Alcoholism per 10,000 pop.	Alcoholics in Treatment[3]	Rate in Treatment per 10,000 pop.	Ratio of Estimated Alcoholics to Alcoholics in Treatment
Urban	3,553,625	445,357	1253	3127	9.0	142:1
Suburban	1,223,834	77,382	632	742	6.1	104:1
Small City	3,889,873	235,086	604	1582	4.1	149:1
Rural	3,136,992	186,186	594	1354	4.3	137:1
Total	11,804,324	944,011	800	6805	5.7	139:1

[1] The complete table is found in Appendix A-2

[2] These figures are based on the Brenner formula, a transformation of cirrhosis deaths. The prevalence of alcoholism in Pennsylvania (1970) as estimated by the Brenner formula is 50% higher than that estimated by the Schaps-Rubin survey, but for the present purposes this does not appear to be a serious threat to the validity of the conclusions.

[3] Since four-fifths of all alcoholics in treatment receive treatment in their county of residence, the numbers of alcoholics in treatment per county was calculated by adding the patient census of the programs located in each county. This will result in some error, since a few patients cross county lines to receive treatment.

contribute to a whole host of deviant behaviors, including alcoholism. On the other hand, they may not have the resources of large cities to grapple adequately with the problem. The present study does not contain the necessary data to test this hypothesis, but it is an issue that is deserving of further study.

It can be inferred from Table 4 that urban programs tend to be larger than those in suburban, small city, and rural counties. For example, while Philadelphia contains only 8.8% of all programs, this city accounts for almost one-fifth of patients in treatment. Conversely, rural areas and small cities tend to have proportionately fewer patients per program as measured by the relative distribution of patients and programs. Further, the mean number of patients per program differs substantially by area. Urban programs have a mean of 130 patients, while small city and rural programs have a mean of 66 and 59, respectively; suburban programs fall in the middle, with 82 patients per program.

As can be seen from Table 6, the proportion of males in treatment who are black far outnumbers the proportion of black males in the population. While less than 10% of the population is black, they comprise almost one-third of the males in treatment. While this over-representation holds true for all areas of the state, there is some difference by population size. In urban areas the proportion of blacks in treatment for alcoholism is about double their proportion in the population, but in areas predominated by small cities, there is a five-fold difference. As pointed out above, there are a number of plausible explanations for this finding. One is that it reflects the higher prevalence of alcoholism among blacks. Another is that blacks are more likely to receive treatment in the kinds of facilities included in the present survey. From the distribution, it can be seen that blacks, both in the general population and in treatment, are located in urban areas. Therefore, at least partially because of residential patterns, blacks tend to be concentrated in large programs.

Finally, we find that most alcohol programs draw their clients from the counties in which they are located; 80.2% of patients in treatment attend programs in their county of residence (see Table 7). This was particularly true for facilities in urban counties. Perhaps owing to the fact that programs in rural and small city areas are relatively few and far between, it is expected that patients will be drawn from several surrounding counties. For instance, it is sometimes the case that two or more counties are combined into a single administrative unit. Many programs in such areas are specifically designed to draw clients from each of the counties comprising the unit, and often establish satellites in these counties. However, virtually all alcoholics in treatment come from Pennsylvania; in all but four counties, 90% or more are from this state. Slightly over one-fifth of all patients are from either of the two major metropolitan areas of Philadelphia and Pittsburgh. (The two

TABLE 6

Number of Male Alcoholics
in Treatment by County Type and Race[1]

County Type	County Population—Male				Males in Treatment			
	White	Non-White	Total	% Non-White	White	Non-White	Total	% Non-White
Urban	1,299,507	381,154	1,680,661	22.6	1270	1260	2530	49.8
Suburban	555,019	33,695	588,714	5.7	434	138	572	24.1
Small city	1,819,515	56,066	1,875,581	3.0	1107	188	1295	14.5
Rural	1,495,455	25,003	1,520,458	1.6	1039	69	1108	6.2
Total	5,169,496	495,918	5,665,414	8.7	3805	1655	5505	30.1

[1] The complete table is found in Appendix A-3

TABLE 7

Place of Residence of Alcoholics
in Treatment, by County Type in Which Treatment Is Received[1]

County Type	No. Alcoholics Treated in This County Type	% from Penna.	% from this country	% from Phila	% from Allegheny Co.
Urban	3127	91.9	88.1	—	—
Suburban	742	93.8	75.1	8.9	0.0
Small city	1582	94.2	67.8	5.4	1.5
Rural	1354	99.3	79.1	0.8	3.1
Total	6805	6446	5458	1451	1597
		94.7%	80.2%	21.3%	23.5%

[1] The complete table is found in Appendix A-4.

cities, located at opposite ends of the state, have virtually no interchange of patients.) But most of these patients are also attending programs in one of the two cities. When programs located in Philadelphia or Pittsburgh are excluded, we find that the number of patients from these cities receiving treatment in other counties is drastically reduced to 4.4% for the former and 1.8% for the latter. Thus, treatment for alcoholism seems to have a strong local base, with only a very few traveling substantial distances in order to receive treatment.

Let us now consolidate this large and diverse body of data on the distribution of patients and programs so that we may arrive at a general picture of the alcoholism problem and the treatment response in Pennsylvania. From Figure 1, it is evident that the treatment programs visited in the present survey tend to be clustered in the two most populous counties, Philadelphia and Allegheny. At the same time, there are large areas throughout the state which have no treatment facilities at all. These gaps can be seen even more clearly in Figure 2, which shows the relative rate of alcoholics in treatment in each county. Twenty-three counties have no alcoholics in treatment.* That this distribution of patients does not reflect need becomes evident when rates of estimated alcoholics across counties are considered (see Figure 3). Alcoholics reside in virtually every county in the state, as estimated by deaths from liver cirrhosis.** In fact, there are several counties having a high prevalence of alcoholism but no alcoholics in treatment. Conversely, a number of counties have low rates of alcoholism but a relatively high number in treatment (see Table 8). When the two sets of rates are correlated to ascertain how well the relative rate of alcoholics in treatment can be predicted from the relative rate of alcoholism in each county, it is evident that, in fact, the latter is not a good predictor of the former (Kendall's $tau_b = .23$). In total, there are only 17 counties out of 67 which have the same relative rate for both alcoholism and alcoholics in treatment (see Figure 4). It would therefore appear that the response to the problem is, for the most part, not guided by its actual prevalence but rather by extraneous factors. If governmental agencies are to allocate scarce monies in the most efficient and appropriate manner, then the factor of prevalence will have to be taken into account. That this has apparently not been the case is evident.

* This is probably not precisely accurate, since a small percentage of alcoholics cross county lines to receive treatment. However, the great majority do not. Thus, for those counties which contained neither a program nor a satellite, it was assumed that there were no alcoholics in treatment.

** Three out of the four counties in which there were no alcoholics, as estimated by the Brenner formula, contained alcoholics in treatment. This apparent inconsistency may be a function of the three-year lag between the prevalence estimate (1970) and the collection of the data on patients in treatment (1973), or it may reflect error in the Brenner formula.

Figure 1

LOCATION OF TREATMENT PROGRAMS

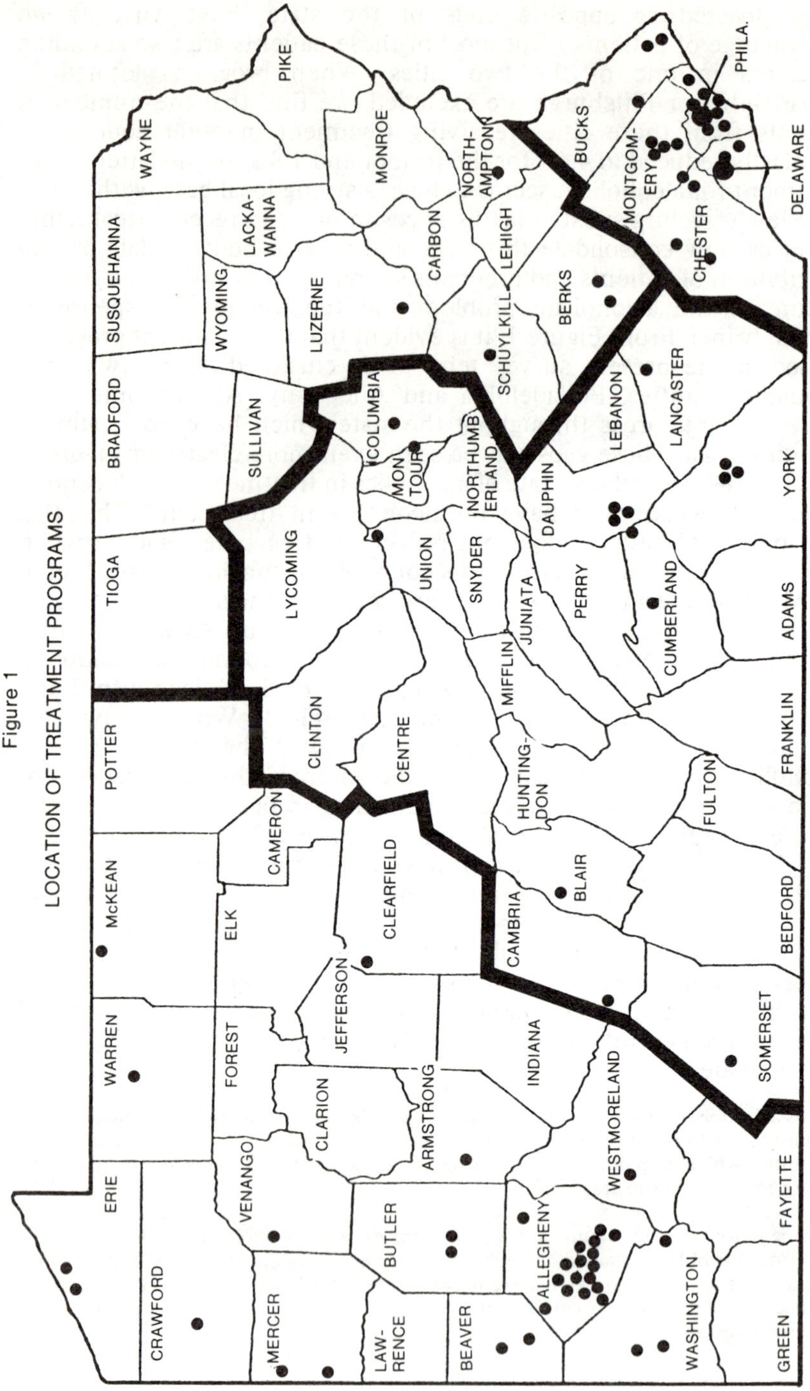

Figure 2

RATE OF ALCOHOLICS IN TREATMENT
PER 10,000 POPULATION

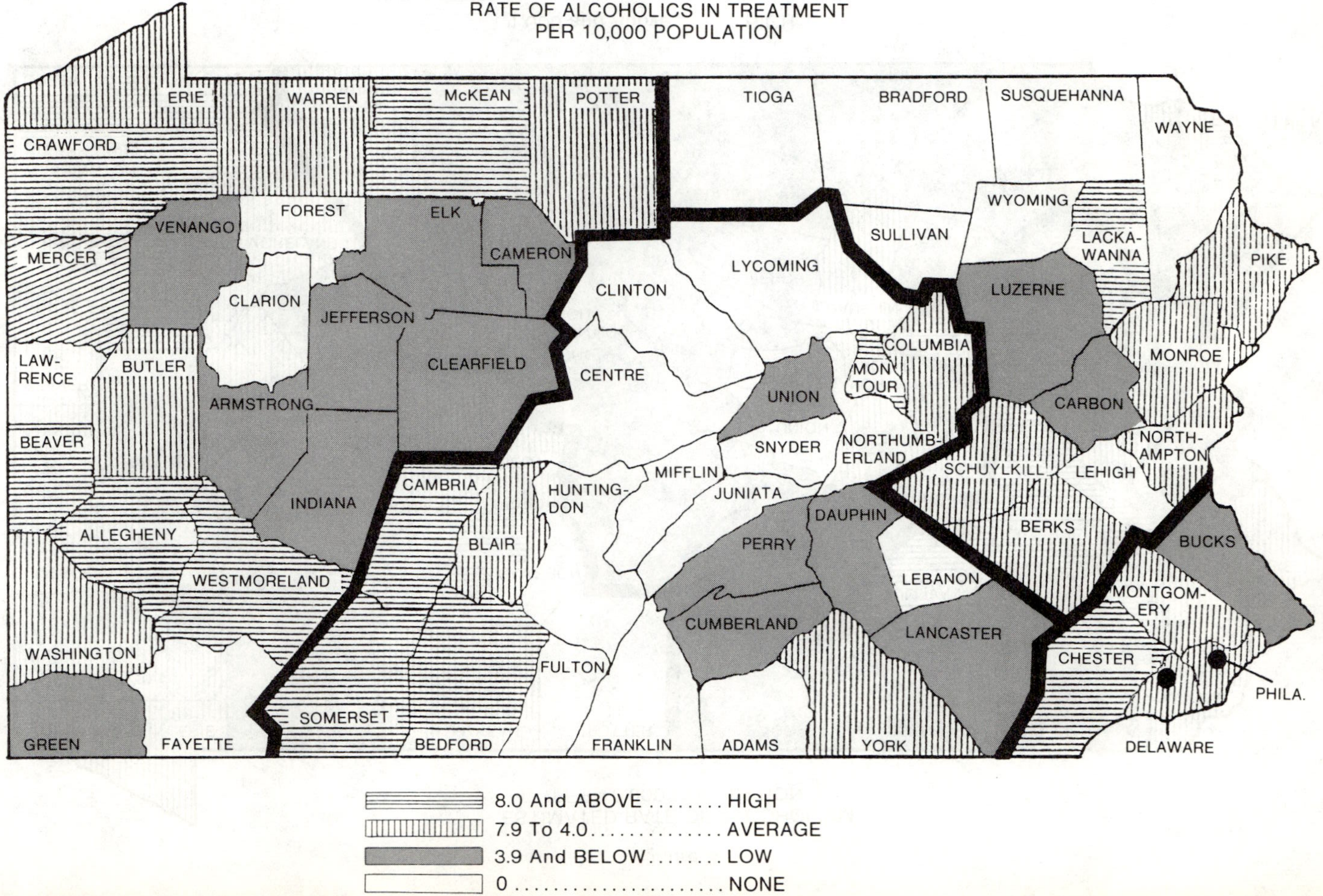

Figure 3

ESTIMATED RATE OF ALCOHOLISM
PER 10,000 POPULATION

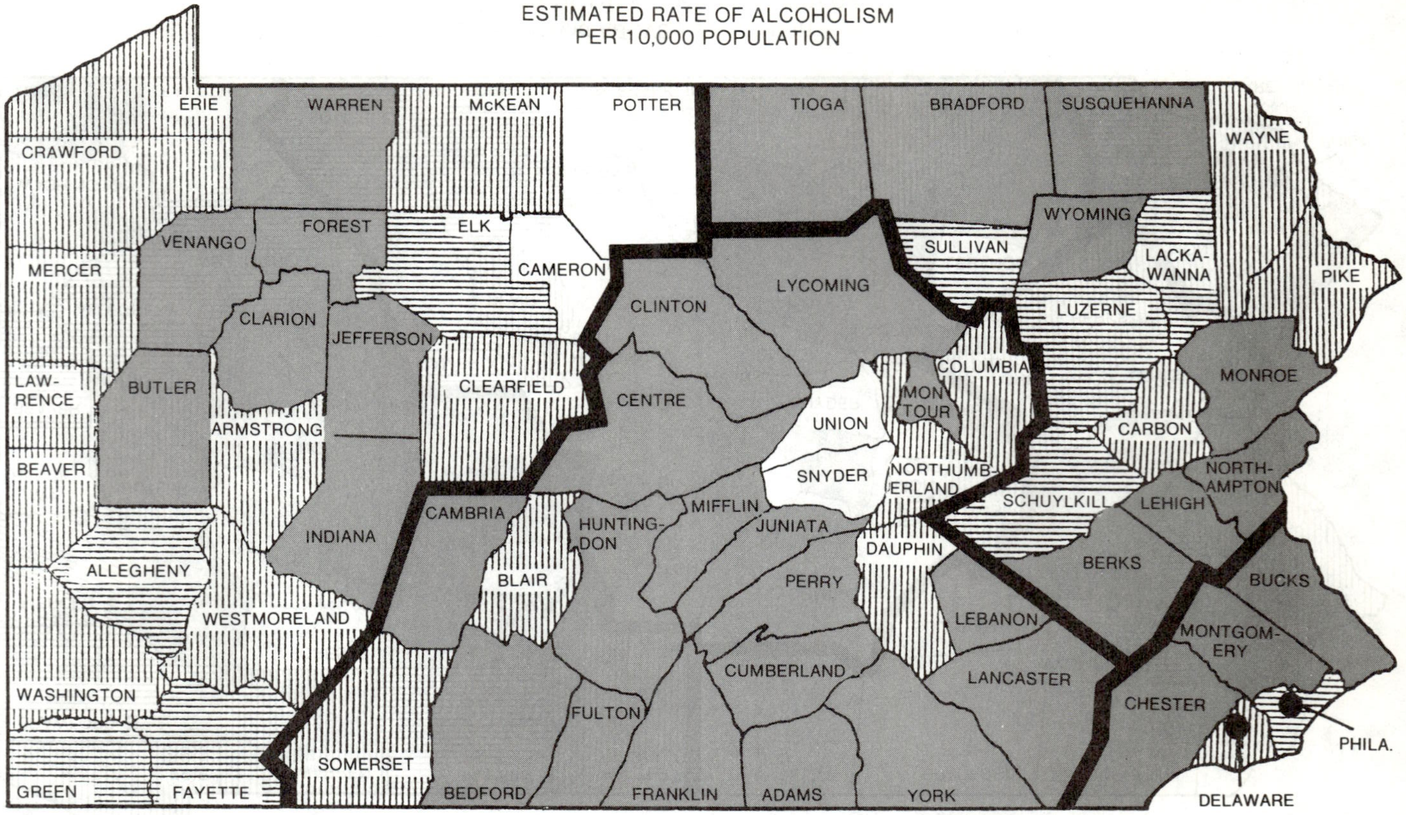

1,000 and Above . . . . HIGH
999 to 600. . . . . AVERAGE
599 and Below . . . . LOW
0 . . . . NONE

1. ESTIMATED BY THE BRENNER FORMULA

COMPARISON OF RATE OF ALCOHOLICS
IN TREATMENT
TO ESTIMATED RATE OF
ALCOHOLISM IN 67 COUNTIES

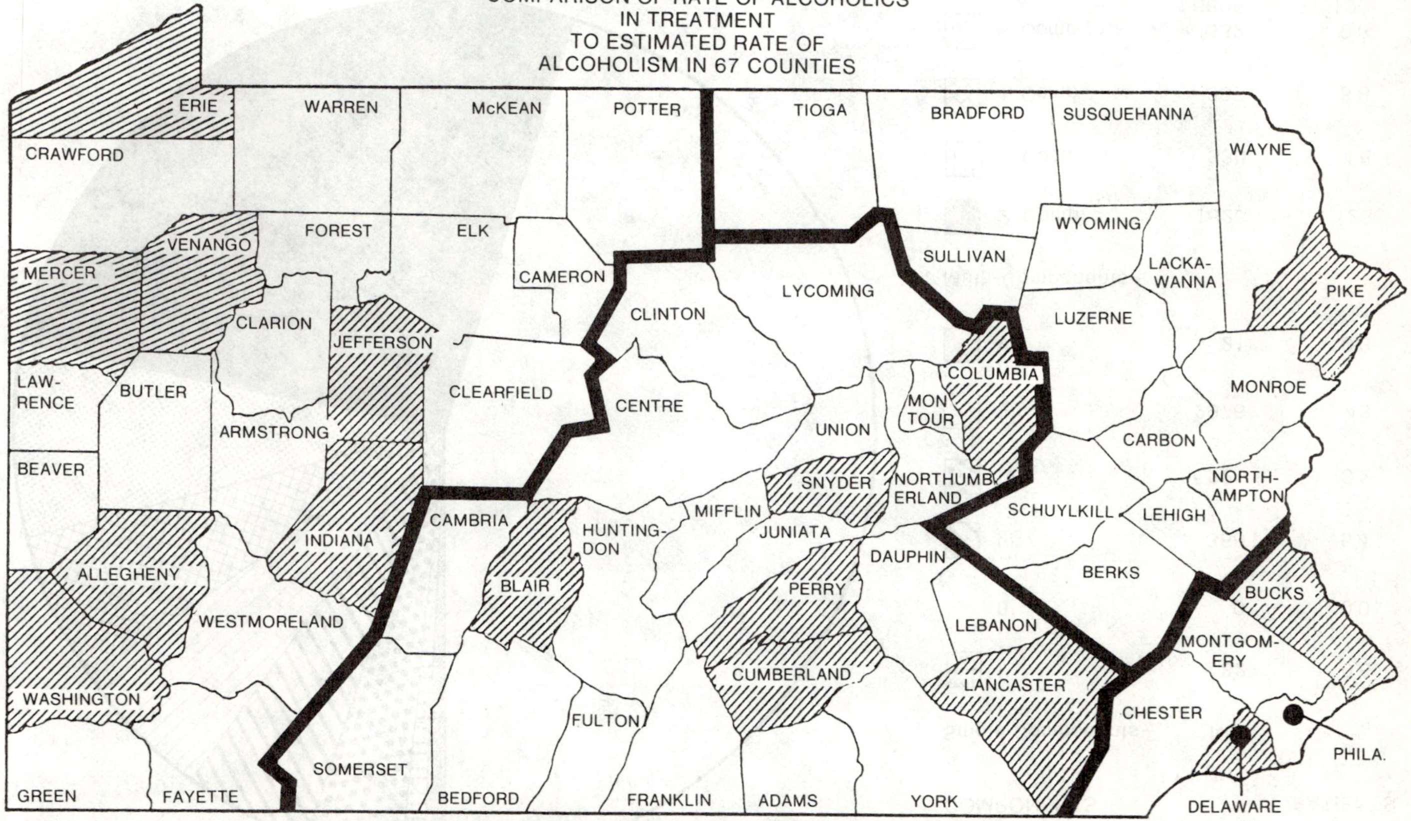

COUNTIES IN WHICH THE RELATIVE RATE OF ALCOHOLISM IS THE *SAME* AS THE RELATIVE RATE OF ALCOHOLICS IN TREATMENT (i.e., COUNTY WITH HIGH RATE OF ALCOHOLISM AND HIGH RATE OF ALCOHOLICS IN TREATMENT ETC.)

COUNTIES IN WHICH THE RELATIVE RATE OF ALCOHOLISM IS *NOT* THE SAME AS THE RELATIVE RATE OF ALCOHOLICS IN TREATMENT.

Figure 5

PATIENT POPULATION BY COMPONENTS

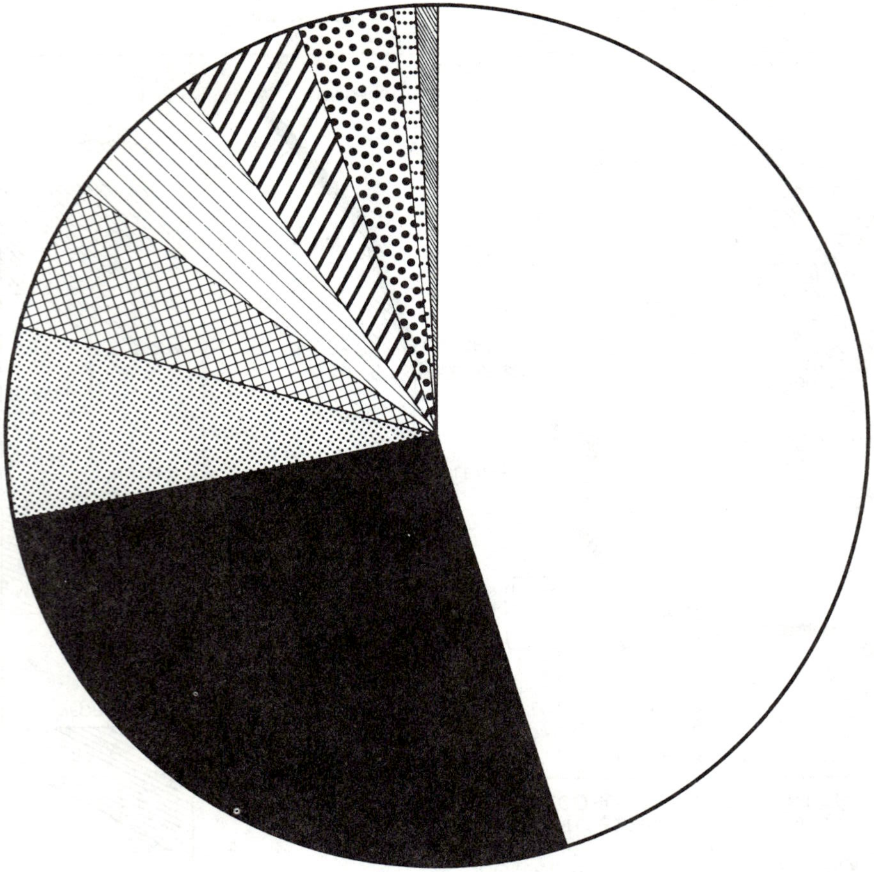

COMPONENTS	PATIENTS	
Single Components—	No.	%
I	32	0.6
II	0	0.0
III	368	5.4
IV	221	3.2
V	2976	43
VI	21	0.3
Multi-Components—		
2. Comp.	1828	26
3. Comp.	330	4.8
4. Comp.	397	5.8
5. Comp.	632	9.3
	6805	100

TABLE 8

Prediction of Rate of Alcoholics in Treatment from Estimated Rate of Alcoholism in 67 Counties

Estimated Rate of Alcoholics per 10,000 Population

	Hi (1000+)	Av (999-600)	Lo (599 & below)	None	
Hi (8.0+)	2	5	4	0	11
Av (7.9-4.0)	2	7	7	1	17
Lo (3.9 and below)	3	4	7	2	16
None	2	3	17	1	23
	9	19	35	4	67

Kendall's $tau_b = .23$

Rate of Alcoholics in Treatment per 10,000 population

Patients and Treatment Types

There is very little variation in types of treatment offered to the alcoholic in Pennsylvania. Out of 6,805 patients in the Commonwealth, 5,557 (81.7%) received treatment as out-patients and 1,248 (18.3%) as in-patients. Almost half of all facilities were comprised of the single element of long-term maintenance, usually on an out-patient basis. Such facilities contained 43.7% of the patients in treatment (see Table 9). The next most frequent encountered program type was the halfway house, which accounted for only 12.5% of the facilities. However, owing to the nature of this form of intervention, in which an environment resembling a private home is provided, it contained only 3% of all patients. In terms of numbers of patients, the second largest treatment type was the dual-element category of detoxification combined with out-patient maintenance care. This type was encountered relatively infrequently, but contained a large proportion of patients.

Males and females were equally represented in most treatment categories. However, males were almost five times more likely to be treated in halfway houses than females. (The male-female difference is much more accentuated among whites than among blacks.) This finding illustrates the pressing need in the Commonwealth for transitional living facilities for women. Further, men were treated in comprehensive five-element programs almost three times more often than females. In general, though, alcoholics in this state, regardless of sex, are most likely to be treated by out-patient community-based facilities, followed by combination detoxification and out-patient maintenance programs.

Black males differed from the rest of the patient population in several respects. Of the four sub-populations, they were the least likely to be treated in either out-patient programs or the programs containing elements I and V. In contrast, they were much more likely than the other groups to be treated in multi-element facilities of the I-II-III-V or comprehensive five-element type. In fact, this latter category was the second most frequent type encountered among black males. At the present, we can only speculate as to the reasons for these differences. One possibility is that black male alcoholics are more likely than any other group of alcoholics to receive treatment under pressure from the criminal justice system.* It is possible that judges may refer them to multi-element programs which tend to be large and well-known. An alternative explanation is that this distribution is geographically determined—both black males and five-element programs tend to be located in urban areas. However, given the overall skewness in the distribution of patients toward treatment type V, regardless of race or sex, inferences about the effect of these two variables on treatment are impossible to make at present.

* 531 or 7.8% of all patients attended alcohol programs under legal pressure. Thus, treatment for alcoholism is largely voluntary.

TABLE 9

Characteristics of Patients in Treatment, by Treatment Type

Treatment Component	Programs No.	Programs %	Patients No.	Patients %	Males No.	Males %	Females No.	Females %	W. Males No.	W. Males %	Non-white males No.	Non-white males %	W. Females No.	W. Females %	Non-white females No.	Non-white females %
I	2	2.5	32	0.6	27	0.5	5	0.4	22	0.6	5	0.3	4	0.4	1	0.3
II	0	0.0	0	0.0	0	0.0	0	0.0	0	0.0	0	0.0	0	0.0	0	0.0
III	9	11.2	368	5.4	281	5.1	87	6.7	256	6.6	25	1.5	76	7.6	11	3.7
IV	10	12.5	221	3.2	210	3.8	11	0.8	188	4.9	22	1.3	9	0.9	2	0.7
V	35	43.7	2976	43.7	2401	43.6	575	44.2	1707	44.3	694	41.9	422	42.0	153	51.7
VI	1	1.3	21	0.3	13	0.2	8	0.6	11	0.3	2	0.1	7	0.7	1	0.3
I,III	1	1.3	14	0.2	13	0.2	1	0.1	11	0.3	2	0.1	0	0.0	1	0.3
I,V	6	7.5	1440	21.2	1044	19.0	396	30.5	828	21.5	216	13.1	329	32.8	67	22.6
III,IV	2	2.5	116	1.7	93	1.7	23	1.8	53	1.4	40	2.4	18	1.8	5	1.7
III,V	1	1.3	100	1.5	90	1.6	10	0.8	90	2.3	0	0.0	10	1.0	0	0.0
III,VI	1	1.3	37	0.5	30	0.5	7	0.5	24	0.6	6	0.4	6	0.6	1	0.3
IV,V	1	1.3	58	0.9	41	0.7	17	1.3	41	1.1	0	0.0	17	1.7	0	0.0
IV,VI	1	1.3	63	0.9	61	1.1	2	0.1	25	0.6	36	2.2	0	0.0	2	0.7
I,III,V	5	6.3	277	4.1	225	4.1	52	4.0	194	5.0	31	1.9	52	5.2	0	0.0
I,V,VI	1	1.3	53	0.8	53	1.0	0	0.0	12	0.3	41	2.5	0	0.0	0	0.0
I,II,III,V	1	1.3	326	4.8	287	5.2	39	3.0	65	1.7	222	13.4	9	0.9	30	10.1
II,III,IV,V	1	1.3	71	1.0	54	1.0	17	1.3	36	0.9	18	1.1	15	1.5	2	0.7
I,II,III,IV,V	2	2.5	632	9.3	582	10.6	50	3.8	287	7.5	295	17.8	30	3.0	20	6.6
Total	80	100	6805	100	5505	100	1300	100	3850	100	1655	100	1004	100	296	100

TABLE 10

Distribution of Alcohol Programs by Area and Treatment Type

Treatment Components	Phila No.	Phila %	Allegheny No.	Allegheny %	Suburban No.	Suburban %	Small Cities No.	Small Cities %	Rural No.	Rural %
I	1	14.3	0	0.0	0	0.0	1	4.2	0	0.0
II	0	0.0	0	0.0	0	0.0	0	0.0	0	0.0
III	1	14.3	0	0.0	0	0.0	5	20.8	3	13.0
IV	1	14.3	3	17.6	0	0.0	5	20.8	1	4.3
V	2	28.5	9	52.9	3	33.3	8	33.3	14	60.9
VI	0	0.0	0	0.0	0	0.0	0	0.0	1	4.3
I,III	0	0.0	1	5.9	0	0.0	0	0.0	0	0.0
I,V	0	0.0	2	11.8	0	0.0	2	8.3	1	4.3
III,IV	0	0.0	0	0.0	2	22.2	0	0.0	0	0.0
III,V	0	0.0	0	0.0	0	0.0	0	0.0	1	4.3
III,VI	0	0.0	0	0.0	0	0.0	0	0.0	1	4.3
IV,V	0	0.0	0	0.0	0	0.0	0	0.0	1	4.3
IV,VI	0	0.0	1	5.9	0	0.0	0	0.0	0	0.0
I,III,V	0	0.0	1	5.9	2	22.2	2	8.3	0	0.0
I,V,VI	0	0.0	0	0.0	1	11.1	0	0.0	0	0.0
I,II,III,V	1	14.3	0	0.0	0	0.0	0	0.0	0	0.0
II,III,IV,V	0	0.0	0	0.0	1	11.1	0	0.0	0	0.0
I-V	1	14.3	0	0.0	0	0.0	1	4.2	0	0.0
Total	7	100	17	100	9	100	24	100	23	100

TABLE 11

Major Secondary Drugs of Abuse Among Alcoholics in Treatment *

Major Secondary Drug	Programs No.	%
Librium	19	23.7
Librium + Valium	18	22.5
Barbiturates	16	20.0
Marijuana	4	5.0
Tranquillizers (unspecified)	3	3.8
Amphetamines	3	3.8
Opiates	3	3.8
Valium	2	2.5
Librium + Stelazine	1	1.2
Librium + Meprobamate	1	1.2
Thorazine	1	1.2
Barbiturates + Tranquillizers	1	1.2
Amphetamines + Tranquillizers	1	1.2
Over-the-counter	1	1.2
None	5	6.5
Don't know	1	1.2
Total	80	100.0

With respect to the relationship between occupational status and treatment, as mentioned above, we found the treatment system to be so dominated by blue-collar workers on the one hand and out-patient maintenance facilities on the other as to make bivariate analysis impossible. However, in general, we found blue-collar workers to be clustered in this treatment category. Owing to the small variation in programs with respect to average occupational level, we were unable to make comparisons across treatment types.

The distribution of programs differed by population density. Urban areas (particularly Pittsburgh) and small cities tended to have a high concentration of halfway houses and out-patient programs (see Table 10). Treatment in rural areas is largely of the out-patient type. Finally, there is no discernible pattern among suburban programs. However, again we found that regardless of area, the treatment of alcoholism was dominated by community-based out-patient clinics.

* Librium® and Valium® are registered trademarks of Hoffman-LaRoche Limited. Stelazine® is a registered trademark of Smith Kline and French Canada Ltd. Thorazine® is a registered trademark of Smith Kline and French U.S. Ltd.

Addiction Characteristics of Patients

Almost three-quarters of the programs in Pennsylvania treat alcoholics who abuse either hard liquor predominantly (32.5%) or some combination of wine, beer, and hard liquor (37.5%). (It has been suggested that the beverage choice of alcoholics does not differ markedly from that of the general drinking population in the same locale.[61]) Over half (55.0%) stated that they would treat either all types of alcoholics or a combination of acute, chronic skid row, or chronic non-skid row alcoholics. Parenthetically, even though there were two detoxification programs, only one of them stated that it treated acute alcoholics specifically. Virtually all of the remaining 35 programs treated chronic non-skid row alcoholics, with only three stating that they treated skid row alcoholics specifically.

There has been much controversy concerning the abuse potential and prevalence of such non-opiates as the barbiturates and the minor tranquillizers, Librium® and Valium®, There is evidence indicating that abuse of these and other drugs is particularly marked among alcoholics.[62-66] In our survey, there was extensive reporting by treatment programs of secondary abuse among alcoholics in treatment. Only five program directors stated that none of their patients was abusing drugs other than alcohol, to the best of their knowledge, and there was no response to this question from another program. Librium,® a combination of Librium® and Valium,® and the barbiturates emerged as the major secondary drugs of abuse (see Table II). While many other drugs or combination of drugs were given, none approached these three in importance. If all responses are combined in which either a major or minor tranquillizer is mentioned, this accounts for almost 60% of the total. When the barbiturates are included, the variation accounted for is increased to almost 80%. Therefore, it appears evident that in many instances the treatment of alcoholism must be directed toward the abuse of several substances of the depressant category, alcohol being perhaps only the *primum inter pares.*

Conclusions

The "average" patient receiving treatment for alcoholism in Pennsylvania is a white male blue-collar worker who attended or graduated from high school, and is in his early 40s. He is being treated on an outpatient basis in a long-term maintenance clinic which is located in his country of residence. He is most likely to be from an urban area, and hence is being treated at a larger program than if he were from a rural, small city, or suburban area. Finally, he tends to abuse either hard liquor or a combination of different types of alcohol, along with secondary abuse of a minor tranquillizer or barbiturate.

The fact that such a typification is possible, general though it may be, is indicative of the homogeneity of both patients and treatment type in the current state of alcoholism treatment. If we are to construct a rational, comprehensive system, several steps are necessary. We must continue to improve and utilize methods of estimating the prevalence of this problem, both in the general population and among its various sub-groups; only in this way can treatment be truly responsive to needs. More attention must be paid to getting the female alcoholic out of residential hiding and into treatment. Rural counties entirely lacking in treatment facilities must be drawn into the system. Finally, the gap which apparently exists in small cities between prevalence and numbers in treatment should be closed.

REFERENCES

1. Edwards, G. Epidemiology applied to alcoholism: A review and examination of purposes. *Journal of Studies on Alcohol, 34:* 28-56, 1973.
2. Popham, R.E. Indirect methods of alcoholism estimation: A critical evaluation. *In:* Popham, R.E. (ed.), *Alcohol and alcoholism,* Toronto: University of Toronto Press, 1970, pp. 294-306.
3. Jolliffe, N. and Jellinek, E.M. Vitamin deficiencies and liver cirrhosis in alcoholism; Part VII, cirrhosis of the liver. *Journal of Studies on Alcohol, 2:* 544-583, 1941.
4. Keller, M. The definition of alcoholism and the estimation of its prevalence. *In:* Pittman, D.J. and Snyder, D.R. (eds.). *Society, culture, and drinking patterns,* New York: John Wiley & Sons, 1962, pp. 310-329.
5. Keller, M. and Efron, V. The prevalence of alcoholism. *Journal of Studies on Alcohol, 16:* 619-644, 1955.
6. Roebuck, J.B. and Kessler, R.G. *The etiology of alcoholism: Constitutional, psychological, and sociological approaches.* Springfield, Ill.: Charles C. Thomas, 1972.
7. Jellinek, E.M. Estimating the prevalence of alcoholism: Modified values in the Jellinek formula and an alternative approach. *Journal of Studies on Alcohol,* 20: 261-269, 1959.
8. Seeley, J.R. Estimating the prevalence of alcoholism: A critical analysis of the Jellinek formula. *Journal of Studies on Alcohol,* 20: 245-254, 1959.

9. Popham, *op.cit.*

10. deLint, J. and Schmidt, W. Consumption averages and alcoholism prevalence: A brief review of epidemiological investigations. *British Journal of Addiction, 66:* 97-107, 1971.

11. Keller and Efron. *op.cit.*

12. Keller, *op.cit.*

13. Terris, M. Epidemiology of cirrhosis of the liver: National mortality data. *American Journal of Public Health, 57* (12): 2076-2088, 1967.

14. Lives and liquor. *Time.* February 4, 1974, p.61.

15. deLint, J. and Schmidt, W. The epidemiology of alcoholism. *In:* Israel, Y. and Mardonis, J. (eds.). *Biological Basis of Alcoholism.* New York: Wiley-Interscience, 1971, pp.423-442.

16. Cahalan, D. and Cisin, I.H. American drinking practices: Summary of findings from a national probability sample; I. Extent of drinking by population subgroups. *Journal of Studies on Alcohol, 29:* 130-151, 1968.

17. Cahalan, D. *Problem drinkers.* San Francisco: Jossey-Bass, 1970.

18. Jellinek, E.M. Phases of alcohol addiction. *In:* Pittman and Snyder, *op.cit.,* pp.356-368.

19. Mulford, H.A. Drinking and deviant drinking, U.S.A., 1963. *Journal of Studies on Alcohol, 25:* 634-650, 1964.

20. Cahalan and Cisin, *op.cit.*

21. Mulford, *op.cit.*

22. Bailey, M.B. Haberman, P.W., and Alksne, H. The epidemiology of alcoholism in an urban residential area. *Journal of Studies on Alcohol, 26:* 19-40, 1965.

23. Terris, *op.cit.*

24. Strayer, R. A study of the Negro alcoholic. *Journal of Studies on Alcohol, 22:* 111-123, 1961.

25. Cahalan and Cisin, *op.cit.*

26. Bailey, *op.cit.*

27. Terris, *op.cit.*

28. Strayer, *op.cit.*

29. Sterne, M.W. Drinking patterns and alcoholism among American Negroes. *In:* Pittman, D.J. (ed.), *Alcoholism.* New York: Harper & Row, 1967, pp.66-69.

30. Cahalan, D. *Problem drinkers. op.cit.*

31. Cahalan and Cisin, *op.cit.*

32. Mulford, *op.cit.*

33. Bailey, *op.cit.*

34. Trice, H.M. and Wahl, J. A rank order analysis of the symptoms of alcoholism. *Journal of Studies on Alcohol, 19:* 636-648, 1958.

35. Terris, *op.cit.*

36. Lisansky, E.S. Alcoholism in women: Social and psychological concomitants. *Journal of Studies on Alcohol, 18:* 588-623, 1957.

37. Cahalan and Cisin, *op.cit.*

38. Mulford, *op.cit.*

39. Terris, *op.cit.*

40. Cahalan and Cisin, *op.cit.*

41. Bailey, *op.cit.*

42. Pearl, A., Buechley, R., and Lipscomb, W.R. Cirrhosis mortality in three large cities. Implications for alcoholism and intercity comparisons. *In:* Pittman and Snyder, *op.cit.*, pp.345-352.

43. Mulford, *op.cit.*

44. Keller and Efron, *op.cit.*

45. Efron, V., Keller, M., and Gurioli, C. *Statistics on consumption of alcohol and on alcoholism.* New Brunswick, N.J.: Rutgers Center of Alcohol Studies, 1972.

46. These data were supplied courtesy of Mr. Frank Ardan, Pennsylvania Department of Health, Office of Birth and Death Records.

47. Schaps, E. and Rubin, E. *A study of prevalence and intensity of drug and alcohol use in the Commonwealth of Pennsylvania.* Prepared for the Governor's Council on Drug and Alcohol Abuse of the Commonwealth of Pennsylvania, August 10, 1973.

48. Lisansky, *op.cit.*

49. Horn, J.L. and Wanberg, K.W. Females are different: On the diagnosis of alcoholism in women. *In: Proceedings of the First Annual Alcoholism Conference,* Washington, D.C.: National Institute of Alcohol Abuse and Alcoholism, D.H.E.W., Pub.No. (HSM) 73-9074, pp.332-354.

50. Lisansky, *op.cit., p.605.*

51. Cahalan, *op.cit.*

52. Trice and Wahl, *op.cit.*

53. Tokuhata, G.K., Digon, E., and Ramaswamy, K. Alcohol Sales and socioeconomic factors related to cirrhosis of the liver mortality in Pennsylvania, *HSMHA Health Reports, 86* (3):253-264, March 1971.

54. Schmidt, W., Smart, R.G., and Moss, J.K. *Social class and the treatment of alcoholism.* Toronto: University of Toronto Press, 1968.

55. Hollingshead, A.B. and Redlich, F.B. *Social class and mental illness.* New York: John Wiley, 1958.

56. Blavis, H.T. and Meyers, W.R. Social class and establishment of treatment relations by alcoholics. *Journal of Clinical Psychology, 22:* 287-290, 1964.

57. Redlich, F.C., Hollingshead, A.B., Roberts, B.H., et al. Social structure and psychiatric disorders. *American Journal of Psychiatry, 109:* 729-734, 1953.

58. Robinson, H.A., Redlich, F.C., and Myers, J.K. Social structure and psychiatric treatment. *American Journal of Orthopsychiatry, 24:* 307-316, 1954.

59. Myers, J.K. and Schaffer, L. Social structure and psychiatric practice: A study of an out-patient clinic. *American Sociological Review, 19:* 307-310, 1959.

60. Barrett, M. *The Pennsylvania state alcohol abuse and alcoholism plan for 1971-1972.* Vol. I: A design for action, Commonwealth of Pennsylvania, Department of Public Welfare, 1972, p.25.

61. deLint and Schmidt. The epidemiology of alcoholism. *op.cit.*

62. Finer, M.J. Habituation to chlordiazepoxide in an alcoholic population. *Journal American Medical Association, 213:* 1342, August 24, 1970.

63. Clare, A.W. Diazepam, alcohol, and barbiturate abuse. *British Medical Journal, 4:* 340, November 6, 1971.

64. Kaufman, A. and Brickner, P.W. Tranquillizer control. *Journal American Medical Association, 224:* 1190, May 21, 1973.

65. Bakewell, W.E., Jr. and Wikler, A. Incidence (of non-narcotic addiction) in a university hospital psychiatric ward. *Journal American Medical Association, 196:* 710-713, May 23, 1966.

66. Bramson, S.M. Abuse of benzodiazepine tranquillizers. *Journal American Medical Association, 225:* 749, August 13, 1973.

Chapter 6

Staff of the Treatment Programs

There may be no greater influence on any professional organization than its staff. Regardless of the expressed purpose of the group, the characteristics of the staff such as size, age, education, and specialization will profoundly affect the organization's development and direction. Nowhere is this more evident than in organizations whose function is to deal with behavioral problems such as alcoholism. While it was beyond the scope of this survey to test this hypothesis in a rigorous manner, one suspects intuitively that the demographic characteristics, division of labor, and areas of specialization of the staff will markedly affect the dominant interests and orientation of such programs. In this light, respondents were asked the race, sex, and educational distribution of the staff, the director's education, and the division of labor, such as treatment, clerical, and so on.

There was a total of 740 full-time and 365 part-time staff members across 80 programs. With respect to distribution by sex, there was a fairly even split (52.6% and 47.4% were males and females, respectively). In terms of race, white staff (76.6%) were clearly predominant over non-white staff (23.4%).

Specialization of Staff

Division of labor among the staff was according to both educational background and function. The main categories according to education were physicians, those with graduate degrees, and college graduates. In terms of function, these three categories were defined as treatment personnel. A fourth category, recovered alcoholics, is neither an educationally or functionally defined position, strictly speaking, but it was assumed that this group would be involved primarily in treatment activities. This category is not mutually exclusive from any of the three educational divisions. Non-treatment personnel generally subserved secretarial, clerical, and custodial functions. In order to understand more fully the staffing of a treatment program, let us briefly describe each position.

Physicians. Doctors serve in several capacities in alcohol treatment programs. Owing in part to the high prestige that this occupation enjoys in our society, physicians are often in leadership positions. Our survey found that almost one-quarter of all program directors were physicians, even though they comprised only 3% of the total full-time staff. This is not to say that physicians receive training that makes them especially well qualified to direct an alcohol treatment program. In fact, the opposite is usually the case, since few medical schools include in their curricula courses either in the treatment of addictive problems or in program administration. However, it is often easier for the program to raise funds, obtain cooperation with the medical community, and receive referrals if the director is a physician. The medical specialties most commonly represented among physician program personnel are psychiatrists and internists. The former often supervise therapeutic activities. The latter are generally utilized to perform routine physical examinations, prescribe tranquilizers, and treat non-alcohol-related diseases, often on a part-time consulting basis (one-third of the part-time staff of programs was comprised of physicians).

Mental Health Professionals. This category encompasses a disparate array of both training levels and specialties, and comprised 40% of the full-time staff. Educational levels ranged from a bachelor's degree to a doctorate, with specialization in such areas as psychology, social work, counseling, and vocational rehabilitation.

Bachelor's degree-level staff are generally utilized for supervised counseling and to aid the patient in contacting various social agencies. Staff members with graduate degrees perform many of the same tasks as lower level mental health professionals, and in addition, serve in a supervisory capacity, conduct in-depth psychotherapy, and handle many of the administration details involved in an alcohol treatment program.[1]

It has been suggested that mental health professionals alone receive the type of training that makes them uniquely capable of treating the alcoholic. Krystal states that "... if we find that practically all emotional problems and psychological syndromes are observable in the problem drinker, we have to provide therapeutic personnel familiar with all of the deviations of mental health."[2] This group includes both mental health professionals—psychologists, social workers, and counselors—and psychiatrists. In addition, non-medical mental health professionals aid not only in dealing with the alleged personality dynamics of alcoholism but also with the problems in social functioning that often accompany and help to label problem drinking. A wide variety of therapeutic activities may be performed, reflecting the specialty of the staff member, including, for example, vocational rehabilitation and family therapy. They represent a vital component in the therapeutic endeavor, since the training afforded to psychiatrists does not tend to equip them to deal with problems in social functioning.

Recovered Alcoholics. This group represents the third major component of treatment personnel. Comprising over one-quarter (27.3%) of the full-time staff of alcohol treatment programs in Pennsylvania, the background and approach which the recovered alcoholic brings to the therapeutic enterprise differ markedly from those of the physicians and mental health professionals. Rather than relating to the individual in terms of healer to patient, the recovered alcoholic offers help in the form of sharing common problems, experiences, and life histories. The practice of recovered alcoholics functioning as lay therapists began in Alcoholics Anonymous, largely as a reaction to the unwillingness of physicians to treat alcoholics. (See Chapter 11.) Virtually all ex-alcoholic counselors are products of this organization.[3]

While this group can make a substantial contribution to the treatment effort, there are potential problems. First, the lack of professional training may result in the commission of serious therapeutic blunders. Second, there is always the danger of relapse of the recovered alcoholic, which would threaten the stability of the entire staff. Third, if the ex-alcoholic counselor maintains too close an allegiance to Alcoholics Anonymous, he may place undue pressure on the client to become a member regardless of the appropriateness of such a course of action. It has been suggested that recovered alcoholics not be used as lay therapists owing to such potential shortcomings, but rather that they would be most helpful in positions involving, for example, community relations and recreational activities.[4] However, it was readily apparent to the survey team that this component of the treatment staff made contributions of a type that could not be duplicated by staff having the accepted professional credentials but lacking in the ability to share the experiences of a common problem. The significance of this contribution is roughly reflected by the correlation between proportion of recovered alcoholics in a program and the quality rating assigned to it by the research team, as is discussed in greater detail in Chapter 10. On the basis of these findings, the research team strongly supports the use of such personnel in the treatment endeavor.

Support Personnel. This category includes secretaries, clerks, and custodians; in other words, those people who do not participate directly in the treatment effort but who nevertheless contribute substantially to the stability of the program. This group comprised 23% of the total full-time staff (secretaries and custodians, 15% and 8%, respectively). The functions of support personnel are myriad, and involve much more than simply filing letters and guarding doors. Often the receptionist is the first line of contact with prospective patients. One of the most common means by which people in need of help are admitted to alcohol treatment programs is by calling in or by having a friend or relative do so. It may well be that the receptionist's ability to deal warmly and sympathetically with the individual, yet collect the necessary preliminary information, is the critical factor in the alcoholic's decision to enter the program. Further, it is generally the secretary's or receptionist's responsibility to keep a daily log of the clients' attendance and to maintain the treatment records in good order. This function has considerable importance, both for research and treatment. Finally, it is the custodian's responsibility to assure that the physical condition of the facility provides a safe, comfortable, inviting setting for treatment, an aspect that is all too often ignored (see Chapter 7).

Director's Training

The educational level and special training of the director of an alcohol treatment program have a substantial impact on it. The director's duties and responsibilities are potentially many, such as performing and supervising clinical activities, serving as chief administrator, raising funds, and acting as a community relations liaison officer. However, the extent to which these functions are either centralized in the director's position or delegated to subordinates is dependent on such factors as the size of the program, the program type, and the inclination of the individual.

From Table 1 it can be seen that there are two main categories of educational background among directors: those with professional training in medicine or one of the mental health specialties, and those with little or no such training. It is likely that in the latter case there is a large proportion of recovered alcoholics who rose to the position of director as a result of their own successful treatment and their desire to help those with similar problems. The rough line of demarcation between the two groups utilized in this study is the possession of a bachelor's degree or above for the professional group and college attendance or below for what is sometimes referred to as the paraprofessional group.* It is clear that the position of director is dominated by the professional group, representing 82.5% of the total.** Directors

* While R.N.'s often do not possess a college degree, they are included in the professional group because of their specialized training.

** Even if all persons at the baccalaureate level and all nurses were excluded, making the possession of a Master's degree the minimum qualification for being a professional, 70% of all program directors would still fall into that category.

TABLE 1

Education of Directors of Pennsylvania Alcohol Treatment Programs

Director's Education	Male	Female	Total
Physician (psychiatrist)	7	1	8 (10.0%)
Physician (non-psychiatrist)	10	0	10 (12.5)
Minister	1	0	1 (1.2)
M.S.W.	14	1	15 (18.8)
M.A. or above	19	3	22 (27.5)
B.S., B.A., B.Div.	6	2	8 (10.0)
R.N.	0	2	2 (2.5)
College attendance	6	1	7 (8.8)
High school attendance	5	1	6 (7.5)
No High school	1	0	1 (1.2)
Total	69	11	80

of alcohol programs are usually professionals and, like the patients they treat, they are predominantly men.

Comparing the distribution in Table 1 with the total distribution of staff by education, it is apparent that physicians and staff with graduate degrees are over-represented in the director's position. While physicians comprise only 3% of the total staff, they represent 22.5% of the directors. Similarly, while only 13.8% of the staff have graduate degrees, almost half (47.5%) of the directors have achieved this level. This is in contrast to the findings for college graduates and below. One-quarter of all staff members are college graduates in comparison to one-tenth of the directors. Further, while 58% of the total staff have less than a college degree, only 20% of the directors are in this group. It may be concluded from these data that directors tend to have disproportionately high levels of training in comparison with staff generally. While this training may not make the individual specifically qualified to run an alcohol treatment program, the social prestige and community contacts that generally accompany advanced education may be viewed as compensating for a lack of special knowledge in the field of alcoholism.

Staffing Patterns by Treatment Component

The functional allocation of staff affords a great deal of information about a treatment program—the intensity of care provided, the types of therapy and services offered, and the general level of activity. While there is considerable variation within components, an aggregate analysis across components provides a broad view of the staffing patterns of alcohol programs from a *systems* perspective.

It is evident that there is much variation across components with respect to both size and specialization of staff. Regarding size, it was found that two-component programs had both the largest and smallest staffs. Programs containing components III and IV had the largest staff, with a mean of 56 per program, while the single program characterized by components I and III had only two staff members. Among the single-component programs, out-patient clinics (V) had the smallest staff, with an average of 3.2 per program; intensive in-patient (III) had the largest, with approximately 16 staff per program. (See Appendix A-5 for a complete breakdown of staff by program type.)

In terms of treatment, it is far more important to analyze the size of the staff relative to the number of patients in the program than to simply show the absolute number of staff. As is discussed at some length in Chapter 10, there is a rough correlation between the staff-to-patient ratio and the quality of the program as evaluated by the survey team. It is probable that, as the number of patients per staff member decreases, both the quantity and quality of attention will increase. From Table 2 it can be seen that in the three categories of treatment personnel, the staff-to-patient ratio is highest among out-patient clinics: 1:27 as compared to 1:9 over all components. In one sense, this is to be expected since this component is intended for patients who are capable of living and working in the community on a full-time basis. Therefore, not as many staff members are required for intervention as would be in the case of detoxification or intensive in-patient programs. However, the discrepancy in the staff-to-patient ratio between component V programs and all other types is so large as to suggest that this difference is not simply a logical outgrowth of its function in the treatment system. Rather, it may be a result of a tendency for serious understaffing in this type of program. It appears that many functions in out-patient clinics are performed by part-time staff (see Table A-5). This program type was one of only four in which the number of part-time staff was greater than full-time staff. This suggests some potentially serious implications in terms of continuity of care and program stability, although this hypothesis cannot be tested from the data collected in our survey. The findings for out-patient clinics are in sharp contrast to those for the other single-component programs. Program types I and III were found to have the lowest ratio of patients to staff while component IV programs had a somewhat higher ratio. This corresponds to the level of intensity of treatment that is characteristically offered in those programs; as the intensity of the therapeutic environment decreases, the number of patients per staff increases. But the drastic increase observed among out-patient clinics is greater than would be expected, given its function. Since this element accounts for half of both the alcohol treatment programs and

TABLE 2

Number of Full-Time Staff and Staff/Patient Ratio by Treatment Component[1]

Component	Total Full-Time Staff[2]		Physicians		Professionals Other Than Physicians		Recovered Alcoholics		Non-Treatment		Patients
	No.	Ratio	No.	Ratio	No.	Ratio	No.	Ratio	No.	Ratio	
I	21	1:2	2	1:16	8	1:4	2	1:16	4	1:8	32
II	0	—	0	—	0	—	0	—	0	—	0
III	143	1:3	4	1:92	49	1:8	56	1:7	38	1:10	368
IV	33	1:7	0	—	9	1:25	14	1:16	5	1:44	221
V	112	1:27	2	1:1488	61	1:49	12	1:248	33	1:90	2976
VI	0	—	0	—	0	—	0	—	0	—	21
2 comp.	230	1:8	6	1:305	92	1:20	47	1:39	62	1:29	1828
3 comp.	78	1:4	5	1:66	15	1:22	7	1:47	19	1:17	330
4 comp.	27	1:15	1	1:397	18	1:22	3	1:132	3	1:132	397
5 comp.	96	1:7	2	1:316	36	1:18	61	1:10	9	1:70	632
Total	740	1:9	22	1:309	288	1:24	202	1:34	173	1:39	6805

[1] This is a summary table. The complete table can be found in Appendix A-5.

[2] Staff categories do not add up to the total full-time staff, since the three treatment categories are not mutually exclusive (i.e. a physician could also be a recovered alcoholic.).

patients in Pennsylvania, this finding is of particular importance.

Let us now turn our attention to the allocation of staff by education and function. Of all the categories, physicians are the most sparsely distributed. The total staff-to-patient ratio is 1:9, while in the case of physicians it is 1:309. Again, there is a high degree of variation across treatment components, with out-patient clinics having the highest ratio (1:1488). The ratio is lowest for detoxification programs (1:16), in all likelihood reflecting the medical setting and orientation of this component.

The findings are similar for professionals other than physicians. Although the variation is not nearly as great as was the case with physicians, out-patient clinics had the highest ratio (1:49) and detoxification programs had the lowest (1:4) as compared to a total of 1:24. The staff-to-patient ratio for professional staff in detoxification programs was the lowest both for all program types and for all categories of personnel. Overall, professionals other than physicians represented the most frequently found category of staff, with a ratio of one such staff member for every 24 alcoholics in treatment. The wide range of educational levels and specialties encompassed in this category may account in part for the finding.

The results for recovered alcoholics, the third category of treatment staff, differ somewhat from the foregoing. Again, out-patient clinics had by far the highest staff-to-patient ratio (1:248), but instead of detoxification programs, intensive in-patient programs (III) had the lowest number of patients per recovered alcoholic staff member (1:7), followed closely by comprehensive five-component programs (1:10).

The fourth staffing category was composed of non-treatment personnel. Here again the findings departed markedly from the composite results. The highest staff-to-patient ratio was found not among out-patient clinics but rather in four-component programs (1:132), specifically of the type comprised of components I, II, III, and V. The lowest ratio was found in detoxification programs (1:8). The somewhat lower relative ratio of non-treatment staff in component V programs as compared to the distribution of other staff categories in this program type may be a reflection of the need of such facilities to have sufficient personnel to maintain the patient records and daily logs. This function may be particularly important in this case, since the patient load is the highest of any component in the treatment system.

Conclusion

Two main conclusions may be reached from the findings on staffing. The first is that the program type that was found most frequently and treated the most alcoholics also had the largest number of patients per treatment staff. A higher staff-to-patient ratio is expected here than in the case of most other components, because it represents a less intensive form of treatment, intended for those who are able to live and work in the community on a full-time basis. However, there is a distinction between staffing that corresponds to function and actual understaffing. Consider the following findings: out-patient clinics had the lowest ratios and also had the lowest relative number of treatment staff; programs with low staff-to-patient ratios received the lowest quality rating. Thus, it is likely that the problem is out-patient clinics lay in the direction of understaffing rather than a functionally determined staffing pattern. A worthwhile area for further research would be to delineate the appropriate staff and corresponding patient size given the function of the program.

The second conclusion is that staff composition varied by program types. Among single component programs, detoxification facilities tend to have a relatively high proportion of professionals compared to the number of patients, while intensive in-patient programs are dominated by recovered alcoholics, many of whom do not have advanced degrees. The problem for the treatment system is to determine what educational background and area of specialization is appropriate for what functions. Only in this way can the staffing pattern of program types be fitted to the needs of the entire system. As was stated in the drug survey:

> *Not all staff members need to have training in all areas of drug abuse treatment. Not every worker must have a B.A. degree. Not every B.A. must have a Masters or Ph.D. degree to be a useful staff person ... administrators must accept the responsibility of differentiating the key positions from those jobs that do not require either great breadth or depth of training. The staff member who gives emergency aid or crisis treatment need not be highly skilled in a professional sense. But he needs to possess some practical knowledge and experience.*[5]

From the perspective of the state government, these findings pose some serious questions about the allocation of personnel. It seems quite clear from the foregoing that merely leaving matters to unaided chance has resulted in some serious problems of staff allocation. While further work is required in terms of developing adequate guidelines on staffing patterns in relation to the service needs of patients, it seems likely that the pool of personnel available to treat problems related to alcoholism will eventually have to be considered as a state-wide resource and will have to be allocated by some means other than chance. In short, the field of alcohol treatment does not appear to be exempt from the problems of maldistribution which are plaguing the field of health manpower generally.

References

1. Adler, F., Moffett, A.D., Glaser, F.B., et al. *A systems approach to drug treatment.* Philadelphia: Dorrance & Co., 1974, pp.119-121.

2. Krystal, H. Who is qualified to treat the alcoholic? II. The advantages of the professional psychotherapist. *Journal of Studies on Alcohol, 24:* 706-712, 1963, p.708.

3. Bacon, S.D. The administration of alcoholism rehabilitation programs. *Journal of Studies on Alcohol, 10:* 1-47, 1949.

4. Bacon, *Ibid.*

5. Adler, et al, *op.cit.,* p.138.

Chapter 7

Facilities

There has been a great deal of interest recently in the influence of the physical environment on human behavior. It is believed that such elements as color, furniture arrangement, room size, and the like profoundly affect both emotions and actions. Particular interest has developed around the issue of environmental effects on mental patients. In the future, it is argued, architects must design such facilities with an understanding of the dynamics of mental illness, so that structure is determined by function.[1-3] The idea is that space should be viewed as a therapeutic resource, in the same way as various verbal techniques and chemical substances are used in the care of the mentally ill. There is no reason to believe that facilities for the treatment of alcoholism should be designed with any less attention to this resource.

In this light, it is safe to say that most of the programs visited in our survey would benefit greatly by more innovative and therapeutic use of space. While few facilities were actually dilapidated, many were drab, cold, and depressing. There was an air of impersonality and gloom that is likely to be anything but helpful to the the alcoholic who is attempting a recovery. While this was not the case with every facility, it was true in a sufficient number of cases to warrant concern.

There was a wide variety of facilities, in terms of building type, size, condition, and location. They ranged from an examining room in a hospital to a beautiful old farm house in the country. Some of the more unusual sites were a warehouse, a convent for the White Sisters of Africa, and a resort hotel. One program was located in a former bordello, complete with appropriate ceiling paintings and ornate wooden moldings. In terms of condition, they range from a suite of modern, cheerful, brightly decorated rooms in a comprehensive health care centre to a few cramped, dark cubicles in the basement of a hospital. In size, the facilities went from one extreme of a 75-room former resort hotel to a single room in an office building.

In virtually all cases, the facility was originally intended for some other completely unrelated purpose and had to be modified to suit the needs of alcohol treatment. As pointed out above, this has often resulted in the unfortunate situation in which structure determines function rather than vice versa. For example, in the case of some out-patient clinics located in hospitals, in order to get to the program it was necessary to travel through long, dimly lit corridors, past operating and examining rooms, with pre-operative patients waiting in the hall. In fact, in one such program, the receptionist in the lobby of the hospital had never even heard of the facility and had no idea where it was located. It is unlikely that such conditions are conducive to recovery. While funding limitations often do not permit major alterations in the physical plant, or optimally, the construction of a new facility for the specific purpose of alcohol treatment, certainly more imagination could be exercised in the utilization of space.

While a wide range of building types is represented in the treatment system, four-fifths of all programs are located in hospitals, former private residences, or office buildings. As can be seen in Table 1, there is little variation across treatment components except for intensive residential programs (Component III) and comprehensive five-component programs. The fact that almost half of all alcoholism treatment facilities were located in hospitals is testimony to the dominance of the medical model in Pennsylvania.

In view of the fact that almost half of all patients are treated in community-based out-patient clinics, it is important to take special note of their physical condition. Most were located in a few rooms of a hospital or office building, often as part of a mental health centre. While few were actually run down, most were unimaginative, sparsely furnished, and somewhat drab. It was often the case that rooms used for individual counseling, which is the major type of therapy in such programs, were cramped and poorly lit, with little visual stimulation. It has often been pointed out that alcohol facilities should have their own entrance in order to decrease the institutional atmosphere and engender feelings of trust.[4] This was rarely the case.

The mediocre condition of most out-patient facilities cannot be attributed to poor or uncertain funding since all but two received the major proportion of their funds from the local, state, or federal

TABLE 1

Location of Programs by Treatment Component[1]

	I	II	III	IV	V	VI	2 Comp.	3 Comp.	4 Comp.	5 Comp.	Total	Percent
Hospital	2	0	4	0	15	1	9	4	2	0	37	46.3
Former Private Residence	0	0	1	7	7	0	1	2	0	0	18	22.5
Office Building	0	0	0	0	9	0	1	0	0	0	10	12.5
Farm	0	0	1	0	0	0	0	0	0	0	1	1.3
Storefront	0	0	0	1	3	0	1	0	0	0	5	6.2
Hotel	0	0	2	2	0	0	0	0	0	1	5	6.2
Other	0	0	1*	0	1†	0	1**	0	0	1††	4	5.0
TOTAL	2	0	9	10	35	1	13	6	2	2	80	100.0

* Old-age home
** Orphanage
† Convent
†† Warehouse

[1] In the small number of cases where more than one location was mentioned, the programs were categorized according to the type of building in which the main or administrative offices were located.

government. While it might be expected that programs having to rely on the vicissitudes of patient fees and contributions would be in the worst physical condition, this was not so. That imaginative, therapeutic surroundings are eminently possible was demonstrated by a publicly-funded program located in a community mental health centre. In addition to the usual number of counseling rooms, there was a large recreation room which was designed to resemble a neighborhood tavern. It was outfitted with ping-pong tables, pinball machines, tables and chairs, and an actual bar where soft drinks were served. Given the population being treated, it was felt that this would provide a familiar, unthreatening environment in which to receive help.

In general, intensive residential programs (Component III) were in the best condition. Generally in suburban or outlying areas of cities, they tended to be located on former estates or farms. The buildings were often large old homes, cared for in part by the residents. The other residential facility, halfway houses, went from one extreme similar to Component III programs to a shabby, dilapidated, boardinghouse atmosphere; there were few in between. The physical plants of the remaining components ran the entire gamut from thoughtful, imaginative use of space to the majority in which the environment was bland in every way, to the few that were entirely unfit for use as treatment facilities.

The geographic location of programs seemed to be a major factor in the variation in physical condition. Although there was a number of exceptions, programs located outside of cities seemed to be in better condition. Regardless of whether they were located in the suburbs, small towns, or rural areas, non-urban programs appeared to make better use of available space. This is particularly evident when comparing programs with the same components located in different areas. For example, as stated above, halfway houses (Component IV) tended to be either in extremely good or extremely poor condition. But it was the case that condition could be predicted by location. All but one of the halfway houses in small towns were described in such terms as "beautiful, large old houses with comfortably furnished, home-like rooms." It appeared that every effort was made to decorate and maintain them in such a way that they resembled a typical, single family, middle income home. Since halfway houses are conceptualized as transitional living facilities between intensive in-patient and community-based out-patient treatment or Alcoholics Anonymous, this homelike atmosphere is appropriate. In contrast, urban halfway houses, all but one of which were located in Allegheny County, tended to be in deplorable condition. In most cases, they were found in rundown areas of the city near factories and warehouses which were adjacent to the central business district. Typically, the houses were shabby with cracked and unpainted walls, dimly lit, sparsely furnished, and often with inadequate heat. They were essentially dormitories.

This atmosphere seems anything but conducive to making a successful re-entry into society.

With respect to most other treatment components, condition could not be predicted as well by location as was the case with halfway houses. An example is out-patient programs; there was little difference by location. Regardless of whether the program was in the central city, the suburban fringe, a small town, or in the middle of a farming area, most Component V programs appeared to take little account of the physical plant. The main difference is that urban programs were almost exclusively located in hospitals and office buildings, while those in other areas were just as likely to be found in former stores, private houses, and community mental health centres. Perhaps there is somewhat more freedom to design facilities in order to implement functions in the latter cases, and in a few instances truly innovative utilization of space was found, but for the most part, non-urban out-patient programs were as unimaginative as urban: adequate but bland. Since such facilities comprise half of all programs and treat half the patients in the Commonwealth, this under-development of an important component is indeed a weakness in the current treatment enterprise.

A final comment on treatment facilities can be made. It has been observed that drug treatment programs are often busy, crowded, seemingly chaotic places.[5] One of the reasons for this is the obvious one of space limitations. While many alcohol facilities were described as cramped, over-crowding did not appear to be a problem. In fact, the opposite was the general rule. The programs were remarkable for their lack of activity. Few patients were seen in or about the facility by the site visit team, even in residential programs. There usually was a receptionist, the program director, and a counselor or two, but no patients. In some instances, there was almost a ghost-town appearance. One explanation for this apparent lack of activity, at least in out-patient facilities, is simply that counseling sessions were not scheduled during the time slot in which site visits were made. However, lack of activity was also the case in a number of residential programs. Even in halfway houses, where patients were somewhat more visible, the level of activity was extremely low; the men seemed to while away the day watching television, reading magazines, and chatting. The highest activity level of any program type was found in the rescue mission (see Chapter 14). Here, most of the residents were actively engaged either in repair work for the thrift shops or the baling operation which supported one of the missions. While the therapeutic value of this work has been debated for many years, at least at the missions there was some sign of actively involved people.

It can be said, of course, that only a few of the alcohol treatment facilities were frankly dilapidated, unsafe for use, or in need of major renovation. In general, they were reasonably adequate from the standpoint of physical safety. However, if the highest quality care is to be provided, mere physical adequacy is not sufficient. It is necessary to utilize to their full potential all existing resources in the therapeutic effort. Not the least of these is the physical environment. Within the limits of space and finances, each facility should be creatively and imaginatively designed in such a way that the environment is a clear reflection of the function of the program and enhances its therapeutic capabilities. In contrast, most of the programs visited were literally depressing to be in, and as a group, seemed to convey through their architectural arrangements a sense of societal condemnation and inevitable doom. The survey team formed a strong impression that the physical environment in which treatment takes place requires significant alteration.

References

1. Watson, D.D., McReynolds, M.D., and Walters, D.B. An evaluation to assist in the development of a city-wide treatment delivery system. Presented at National Conference on Evaluation in Alcohol, Drug Abuse and Mental Health Programs, Washington, D.C., April 2, 1974.

2. Adler, F., Moffett, A.D., Glaser, F.B., et al. *A systems approach to drug treatment.* Philadelphia: Dorrance & Co., 1974.

Chapter 8

Relationship with the Community

In order to present a complete picture of the treatment of alcoholism in Pennsylvania, it is important to describe not only the internal characteristics of treatment programs but also their relationships with the larger world beyond their doors. No treatment enterprise exists in a vacuum. The community is depended upon to fulfill a wide range of program needs, from providing funds to lending garden equipment. In turn, the community should view the program as a readily available resource to deal with the ever-present problem of alcoholism. The research team felt it desirable to measure the degree to which this potentially reciprocal relationship was actually realized. Each program was asked to describe in an open-ended fashion the nature and extent of its contact with four key elements of the community: its immediate neighbors, the police, the medical profession, and the government.

In general, the responses were overwhelmingly positive. In no case did less than three-quarters of the respondents state that their relationship with any of the community elements was other than "good," "excellent," or in some way mutually beneficial. In what follows, the nature of the relationship between the treatment enterprise and the community in the Commonwealth of Pennsylvania will be described in greater detail.

Neighbors

Neighbors were defined in a variety of ways, depending on the housing situation of the program. If the program was located in a hospital, other departments and units were referred to as neighbors. In contrast, if it was situated in a commercial area, as was the case with a number of community-based out-patient facilities, the adjacent shops were regarded as neighbors. Finally, programs found in residential areas defined their neighbors as the surrounding homes or farms. In other words, the programs were instructed to define as neighbors any person or group found in the immediate locale of the facility.

The research team did not expect the overwhelmingly positive response given to this question. Out of 80 programs, 72 (90%) stated that their relationship with neighbors, defined as above, was "good," "excellent," "friendly," and so on. A common response was that at the inception of the program, the neighbors expressed misgivings at the least, and at times outright hostility. One respondent described an incident in which the driveway leading into the facility was blocked by a telephone pole that his neighbor had taken care to chop down. The director of a halfway house stated succinctly, "The neighbors were ready to lynch us." However, with the passage of time, most of the neighbors were apparently able to acclimate themselves to the presence of the programs. This finding was particularly the case with programs located in residential areas. It was often reported that once the initial "fear of the unknown" was overcome, both the program and the neighborhood residents were able to interact in a mutually friendly manner, extending assistance to one another when needed. This may be evidence that the stigma of alcoholism is finally being removed and that people are beginning to learn to regard the alcoholic in treatment as a neighbor and legitimate member of the community rather than a pariah.

It is indeed ironic that in every instance of a reportedly poor relationship with the immediate neighbors, the program was located in a hospital. While only 5% of the overall responses were negative, the homogeneity of the settings in which these negative responses occurred was striking. For a social problem that many people have striven for years to have classified as a disease, it is deeply meaningful that hospitals provided the *least* congenial atmosphere for its treatment. However, in fairness, it must be stated that out of the 37 programs located in hospitals, 30 reported positive relationships with their neighbors. (Three stated that they had little contact with other units in the hospital.) The relationship of alcoholism treatment programs with the medical community in general will be discussed at some length below.

Police

The relationship of treatment programs with the police, both state and local, was the most positive of any of the four community elements. Favorable relationships were reported by 94% of the programs, while only 4% (three programs) stated that their experience with the police had been poor. (Two programs reported no contact with the police.) This is a very encouraging finding, since it is often the case that the police are the first line of contact in dealing with the alcoholic. If there is not ready understanding and cooperation between programs and police, the revolving-door method of dispensing justice to the public inebriate is likely to be fostered. Fortunately, however, the positive and informal relationship that was overwhelmingly reported in the present survey would indicate that the police are willing to make use of local treatment facilities, rather than simply deposit the individual in the drunk-tank for the night, only to release him the next day. Hence, legislation which would encourage this practice and provide for it a sound legal basis, such as the proposed Public Inebriate Law (Appendix C), is likely to have considerable positive impact.

Programs related to the police in a variety of ways. For instance, a number mentioned that they had organized lecture series to inform the local police force about the nature of alcoholism. Others reported that the chief of the local force was active in mental health affairs. One multi-component program had a police pick-up system, in which the police notified the program as soon as someone was brought to their attention for public drunkenness. The program and the police then picked up the individual jointly, and in the great majority of cases brought him to the treatment facility, whereupon he was diagnosed, evaluated, and assigned to a treatment component. In one community, people arrested for public drunkenness were paroled into the custody of program counselors. Several respondents mentioned that they had "earned" good rapport with police because the latter used the program as a dumping ground for drunks. While this perhaps implies exploitation on the part of police, the programs recognized that dumping public inebriates in a treatment facility is far more desirable than imposing a one-night jail sentence.

Medical Community

The medical community for a given program was defined as the hospitals, clinics, and private physicians which existed in sufficiently close proximity that they could conveniently be utilized by the program. The pattern of responses indicated that of the four community elements, the relationship between programs and the medical community was the most negative. Less than three-quarters (73%) of the respondents stated that their relationship with the entire medical community was good, as compared to virtually unanimously positive replies with respect to immediate neighbors and the police. While it is true that the majority of programs enjoyed good relationships with this element of the community, their enthusiasm was tempered in a number of cases by the feeling that the actual nature of the association was one of benign neglect on the part of the medical community rather than active support. As one respondent stated, "Things are touch and go, but we may make it with them."

Another 9% reported that the program's relationship was good with some elements of the medical community, but poor with others. In most of these instances, the respondent specified that the trouble lay with private physicians. They stated that such physicians tended to ignore the programs' attempts at forging a reciprocal relationship and in extending information to hospitals and physicians about alcoholism.

Almost one-fifth (18%) asserted that they had negative experiences as a rule with local physicians and hospitals. Common complaints were difficulties in finding beds for detoxification, lack of referrals to programs by hospitals and physicians, and a general unwillingness to treat the alcoholic. At the same time, bitterness was also expressed toward the practice on the part of some physicians of using the program as a dumping ground. When the police did this it was viewed as beneficial, but in the case of physicians the practice was regarded as a ploy to escape having to deal with the alcoholic.* In a few instances, physicians were deeply resented for prescribing what was thought by respondents to be excessive doses of barbiturates and tranquillizers. It was felt that this was yet another means that physicians used to send the alcoholic quickly on his way. As one program director stated, "Physicians in this county are the biggest pushers, and they do it legally, particularly with alcoholics."

As mentioned, there is a marked tendency for programs located in hospitals to have poor relationships with other units in the hospital and the medical community in general. Out of 14 programs reporting negative associations with the medical community, six were located in community hospitals and three in state hospitals. This is somewhat unexpected, since it might be assumed that proximity to medical personnel would engender greater understanding and cooperation. However, the opposite seems to have been the case.

It appears that the widespread acceptance of the disease concept of alcoholism which has been striven for over the past 40 years by pioneers in the treatment of alcohol abuse has not completely filtered down to private physicians and community hospitals. This is ironic because the disease concept, as the term implies, is essentially a medical model. The campaign for the acceptance of this conception of alcoholism was aimed particularly at the medical profession. It was hoped that if the conception of alcoholism as a moral failing could be replaced by the morally neutral disease model, physicians and hospitals would open their doors to the alcoholic. The fact that three-quarters of the programs in the present survey enjoyed a positive relationship with the medical community may be testimony to the success of this

* This is not as contradictory as it may seem. Programs tend to view police generally as having no significant role in the management of alcoholism other than quelling disturbances and occasionally dealing with criminal acts associated with alcohol abuse. Physicians, on the other hand, are viewed as *potentially* capable of making an important contribution to the long-term management of alcohol-related problems.

strategy. But the fact that one-quarter did not may reflect the inherent inadequacy of the disease concept of alcoholism as much as any other factor. However, it is evident that the health professions, particularly physicians, must continue to be educated to regard the alcoholic as an appropriate and worthwhile target at which to aim a treatment effort to which they can significantly contribute, whether or not the disease concept is accepted. It is necessary, for example, for medical students, practising physicians, and other health professionals to receive training on the diagnosis and treatment of alcoholism in order to put an end to the avoidance and rejection that many problem drinkers have encountered in seeking help. There is some indication that the importance of this area is beginning to be recognized by progressive medical and nursing schools.

Government

The role of government, on all levels, is becoming increasingly important in the treatment of alcoholism. Under the provisions of the so-called Hughes Act, which became law in 1970 (see Appendix C), governmental administrative and funding agencies on both the state and federal levels have come into being. In the Commonwealth of Pennsylvania, the state government has directed the creation of county level agencies whose duties and responsibilities in the localities are analogous to those of the single state agency on the state level. In view of these developments, it was surprising that 10 out of the 80 programs (12.5%) had no contact with government. This represented the highest proportion of any community element with which the programs had no relationship. Of the 70 that reported a relationship with government, 50 (83%) stated that it was positive. The most common response was that the primary locus of contact was on the county level, particularly with the office of Mental Health and Mental Retardation. Several others reported that they had frequent contact with county commissioners and received referrals from local magistrates. Three respondents stated that they had a good relationship with local government but a poor one on either the state or federal level. While local officials could be contacted frequently and informally, several program directors reported difficulty in cutting through bureaucratic red tape at higher levels.

Of the four community elements, programs reported the second highest proportion of poor relations with government. Nine programs (13% of programs having contacts with government) stated that they had negative experiences with this element. Two-thirds of those with a poor relationship reported that for the most part the problem was on the local level, although no level of government had been particularly helpful. Commonly reported problems were that little cooperation had been extended by various local agencies concerning funding; programs were not asked for their input in the formation of policies that directly affected them; and there was a felt lack of communication between programs and agencies. For example, one program threatened to relinquish its funding and close rather than participate in a county plan that the director stated he had no part in devising. While most programs did not take this extreme position, there was a definite feeling among a number of programs that government on all levels was indifferent, rigid, or actually hostile.

Conclusion

The results of the present survey indicate an overwhelmingly positive relationship between the treatment enterprise and the community. In all cases, a majority of programs stated that their contacts with the four elements of the community under study were good, mutually beneficial, and cooperative. It is to the credit of all concerned that such generally satisfactory relations could be forged in a situation which is potentially difficult. It is perhaps the case that alcoholism treatment programs might survive without the understanding and support of the community. At the same time, since no community is immune to the problem of alcohol abuse, it can ill afford to be without ongoing, high quality treatment. Thus the benefits of forging such cooperative interaction are many.

However, this is not to say that all contacts between programs and the community have been perfectly harmonious. As the responses to the interview indicated, this is far from true, particularly with respect to the medical community and the government. These are two highly critical community elements with respect to the management of alcoholism. While relationships here are generally good they are of such importance that this is not sufficient. Unless there exists throughout Pennsylvania a positive, efficient, and mutually satisfactory relationship between the alcoholism treatment effort, the medical community, and the government, truly adequate treatment will not be forthcoming. This study suggests that such a relationship does not now exist.

Chapter 9

Recommendations from the Programs

In order to construct a viable treatment system which is responsive to patient needs, it is a necessity that there be input from treatment personnel. It is at this level that felt needs are quite concrete and weaknesses in the system are acutely perceived. While government administrators and researchers tend to have a general, global conception of needs, personnel involved directly in the treatment effort are in a position to be aware of specific, tangible requirements. Unless government administrators are sensitive to this input, a truly responsive system is impossible.

This survey requested recommendations only from program directors. Ideally it would have been desirable to have input from every individual directly involved in treatmnet. A survey of drug treatment programs in Philadelphia suggests that personnel on all levels can contribute valid perceptions of the therapeutic process.[1]

Since the creation of the single state agency which is responsible for overseeing both treatment policy and program operation, substantial headway has been made in terms of the creation of the permanent, ongoing treatment system for alcoholism. However, that this systematic perspective had not at the time of the survey completely filtered down to the level of individual programs is illustrated by the

TABLE 1

Recommendations for Alcohol Programs

	No.	%
Treatment facilities (a greater number and more variety)	58	72.5
Funding (more and innovations in funding mechanisms)	30	37.5
Staffing (more and better trained)	19	23.8
Education and prevention (from elementary grades on up; publicity)	35	43.8
Coordination and standardization (coordination of effort on local level; uniform data collection; treatment standards)	29	36.3
Criminal justice system (ending "revolving door")	13	16.3
Evaluation (follow-up and research)	12	15.0
Industrial programs (treatment, training, insurance)	10	12.5
Treatment priorities (more attention paid to alcoholism)	3	3.8

directors' recommendations (see Table 1). Three-quarters of the responses were in terms of the specific treatment needs of particular programs. In addition, one-quarter and over one-third of the recommendations were addressed respectively to staffing and funding problems, which are also program-specific. In contrast, only one-third of the respondents mentioned the need for more coordination and standardization in the system. Further, less than one out of every seven respondents expressed a need for patient follow-up, evaluation, or research. But if the Commonwealth is to construct and maintain high quality service, this component is essential and must be recognized as such.

In order to communicate adequately the felt needs of the system, it is necessary to describe in some detail the nature of the recommendations. These will be presented as they were given and without specific critical commentary.

Treatment Facilities

Of all the recommendations which they offered, program directors were most concerned with the type and quality of existing facilities. Three-quarters of the respondents mentioned this aspect of the treatment enterprise. For the most part, they seemed to be reacting to the lack of particular types of facilities in their communities.

There was a wide range of responses in this category, including the need for more vocational rehabilitation, high quality community outpatient clinics, residential facilities as an alternative to incarceration, and cooperation of hospitals in providing emergency care for alcoholics. Several responses emerged as major themes, specifically the severe shortage of detoxification facilities, halfway houses, and facilities of all sorts to serve the needs of female alcoholics. These three responses were encountered so frequently that it may be safely assumed that the needs are felt throughout the Commonwealth and are not specific to any one location. Since both detoxification facilities and halfway houses—each at different ends of the intervention spectrum—are vital to a comprehensive treatment enterprise, considerable attention must be paid to their development.

The need for detoxification facilities was further emphasized when the directors were asked how many beds were available in community hospitals for this specific purpose. It was found that in the entire Commonwealth less than 500 beds were designated to serve this purpose, including the two programs in which this is the major element of treatment. While many stated that beds were available as needed, it would appear necessary to have a great many more detoxification beds on a permanent, ongoing basis. Residential detoxification programs may be of considerable assistance.

Finally, the need to induce more female alcoholics to enter treatment, which was mentioned in an earlier chapter, emerged as a major theme. Specifically, the lack of halfway houses for women was reportedly presented as a seriously unmet need. While the need for this type of intervention was found to exist for alcoholics in general, only five out of the 10 halfway houses contained women patients, and only one was intended exclusively for women. The remaining five treated males only and would not accept a female alcoholic. If the treatment system is to be responsive, it must take steps to insure that women are afforded the same range of treatment alternatives available to men.

Funding

Over one-third of all programs expressed concern with funding. While some felt that funding was not sufficient, a large number were more interested in the mechanisms for funding rather than the amount. For example, several mentioned that the current pay schedule for medical aid was unrealistic, especially for detoxification; compensation should extend over a longer period of time than is currently the case in order to fully cover the detoxification process. Another suggestion was that either the state or industry should institute insurance coverage for out-patient care, thereby protecting the individual from both the economic burden of treatment and the stigma of the public dole.

Staffing

Related to recommendations concerning treatment facilities is the need for staff development. This was mentioned by one-quarter of the respondents. The most frequently encountered response was the need for more and better-trained staff. It was felt that with a larger number of staff, programs would be enabled to offer a broader range of services, particularly outreach and follow-up. Another suggestion was that state-sponsored training programs be developed in which certification of graduation would be a requisite in order to treat alcoholic patients. This would help to promote a uniformly high quality of care throughout the system, regardless of program type or geographical area.

Education and Prevention

The need to provide information concerning alcoholism to all groups in the population, from elementary school children to nurses and physicians, was regarded as a major goal by almost half of the respondents. Since drinking—within a vaguely delineated range—is a socially accepted and even encouraged behavior, it is deemed essential to inform people of its potential dangers. The emphasis is not on abstinence but rather on socialization into responsible drinking habits. In addition, it was considered important to dispense information on the physiological effects of alcohol, primarily as a means of discouraging drunken driving. Education must begin in the early grades and continue through high school, according to the respondents. In addition, there must be massive advertising campaigns to make the general public aware of the symptoms of alcoholism, the types and locations of available treatment, and the dangers of drunken driving. Further, the respondents strongly recommended that courses on the diagnosis and treatment of alcoholism be included in the curricula of medical and nursing schools. Many felt that the inability of some physicians to recognize the symptoms of alcoholism and their tendency simply to prescribe tranquillizers as the only treatment intervention when symptoms were recognized must be ended. Also, physicians should be made aware of the treatment alternatives that exist in their communities.

The corollary of education is prevention. If the public is educated as to the dangers of alcoholism, the expectation is that problem drinking will decline. It was considered important to remove the stigma from alcoholism and treat it as an addictive disease. The belief that alcoholism is grounded in the social structure and that in order to put an end to alcoholism it is necessary to make radical changes in society was seldom heard. (The response that came closest to this was the suggestion to close all liquor stores.) Rather, it was widely believed that information disseminated in an effective manner would change attitudes toward alcohol consumption and that this would be sufficient for prevention. In general, it was believed that by initiating programs in the schools and embarking on advertising campaigns the goal of prevention would be achieved.

Coordination and Standardization

Recommendations in this category were directly aimed at the treatment system *quo* system. The fact that only one-third of the program directors mentioned systematic recommendations is indicative of the current low level of awareness that a coherent system exists, or ought to exist. Suggestions in this category were directed at coordination of effort both between programs and between government agencies and programs. Several respondents suggested that programs in the same area must engage in the cooperative relationship, in terms of information exchange and program referral. Some stated that there should be a system of central intake, in which patients would be channeled to particular types of treatment, according to their own needs, thereby eliminating inter-program competition. Not only was there a felt need for coordination on the local level, but also there was a desire for an ongoing, well-defined relationship with the single state agency. Such recommendations frequently took the form of routinized mechanisms for program-to-agency input, standardized guidelines for treatment programs, system-wide data collection, and technical assistance. As one program director stated, "We have everything we need; it's just a matter of coordination."

Criminal Justice System

While only 16% of the responses were directed at the criminal justice system, they were all virtually identical in content. Essentially, the message was that alcoholics must be removed from the "revolving door." Throwing public inebriates into the "drunk tank" overnight, it was felt, serves only to create new problems and aggravate old ones. The suggestions which were made included court referrals to detoxification and residential programs, prison programs for alcoholics, and treatment and education for persons convicted of drunken driving. There was also a felt need for greater cooperation and communication between treatment programs on the one hand and the courts and law enforcement on the ohter (see Chapter 8). In general, there was a strong feeling that the inclusion of public inebriates in the criminal justice system was at best inappropriate and at worst a threat to the individual and society.

Evaluation

Included in this category is the need for program evaluation, patient follow-up, and research into alcoholism. It is perhaps indicative of the traditional animosity between the treatment and research enterprises that only 15% of the program directors expressed a concern for research and evaluation. It is sometimes felt by clinicians that research is just another form of government harrassment, bearing no relevance to the treatment effort. However, there was a number of suggestions to the effect that systematic evaluation of programs could serve to improve services. In addition, one respondent expressed an interest in more research on dual addiction. Perhaps the most prevalent response in this category was the need for funds and staff for patient follow-up. Without this component, it was emphasized, the actual efficacy of treatment remains in question.

Industrial Programs

There was some interest (expressed by more than 10% of the respondents) in the role of private industry in alcohol treatment. Their suggestions included insurance programs to finance treatment for alcoholic employees, job programs for alcoholics recently out of treatment, and most frequently, treatment programs in industry. There is reason to believe that industry will be assuming an increasing role in the care and education of alcoholic employees, as is discussed in Chapter 12.

Treatment Priorities

Three respondents expressed the concern that alcoholism was receiving short shrift in comparison to drug addiction, both on a county and state level. It was pointed out that the prevalence of alcoholism was many times greater than that of heroin addiction, and hence should be given more attention by government agencies.[2] However, that this was not a major concern among program directors was illustrated by the fact that only 3.8% of them mentioned this in their recommendations.

Conclusion:

Unless policy-makers are sensitive to the concrete needs of treatment programs, there can be no functional system. In fact, a number of respondents expressed feelings of isolation and powerlessness with respect to decision-making bodies and were relieved to have the opportunity of airing their thoughts to a group of people who were representing, albeit indirectly, the single state agency. In order for the treatment system to survive, there must be routine mechanisms for tapping the needs and recommendations of programs in local communities. To the credit of the single state agency, steps have been taken to achieve this goal, but continual care must be taken to insure the responsiveness of the system to local needs.

On the other hand, one cannot fail to be impressed by the largely parochial nature of the concerns expressed in these recommendations. With few exceptions they related only to the immediate needs of the respondent's particular programs. It was the team's impression that if all of the individual programs had been functioning smoothly, most respondents would have been hard pressed to come up with recommendations of any kind. Essentially similar conclusions were reached in a study of drug abuse programs.[3]

Thus it is clear once again that the notion of a coordinated and systematic approach to all aspects of that complex problem labeled "alcoholism" is not prevalent among practitioners. Leadership in promoting this notion will have to come from outside the treatment area, and very likely from the single state agency. Moreover, there is a strong suggestion that movement taken in this direction may not be since, in the minds of the respondents to this survey, considerations of the moment tend to outweigh all others. Hence it will be the task of the single state agency to assuage pressing and immediate needs while not losing sight of the overall goals of systematic and comprehensive treatment.

References

1. Watson, D.D., McReynolds, M.D., and Walters, D.B. An evaluation to assist in the development of a city-wide treatment delivery system. Presented at National Conference on Evaluation in Alcohol, Drug Abuse and Mental Health Programs, Washington, D.C., April 2, 1974.

2. Glaser, F.B. and Greenberg, S.W. Relationship between treatment facilities and prevalence of alcoholism and drug abuse. *Journal of Studies on Alcohol, 36:* 348-58, March 1975.

3. Adler, F., Moffett, A.D., Glaser, F.B., et al. *A systems approach to drug treatment.* Philadelphia: Dorrance & Co., 1974.

Chapter 10

An Approach to the Quality of Treatment

Introduction

An assessment of the quality of treatment for problems related to alcohol was not a primary goal of this research. Its primary goal was, rather, to describe the nature and location of the intervention effort in the Commonwealth and the numbers and types of individuals with whom that effort was dealing. Yet there was good reason to pay at least some attention to the quality of the intervention effort.

Previous studies of the quality of treatment for alcohol problems and related difficulties in Pennsylvania and elsewhere, though few in number, suggested that problems related to quality might exist. The recent study of drug abuse treatment programs in Pennsylvania had suggested that fewer than one-third of all programs were of good quality, and that less than a quarter of all patients in treatment were receiving care in these programs.[1,2] Preliminary reports of a statewide survey of alcoholism treatment programs in Alaska, although conducted with a dissimilar methodology and applied at the time of the report only to a single program, also revealed problems with the quality of treatment:

> *The results of the chart audit indicate that patients were assigned to treatment methods without a thorough evaluation of their problems and without a recorded assessment of severity and were allowed to progress without follow-up or*

reassessment. . . . The records of this agency are not unique. Other agencies currently being investigated show similar and, in some cases, more discouraging results. Choices of treatment continue to be made with little evidence for the reasoning involved in the selection.[3]

While these results indicated that attention to quality of treatment was in order, the survey team's approach to quality immediately encountered a major methodological problem. The ultimate indicator of quality of treatment is the outcome of treatment. Beyond much argument, those programs are of highest quality which most consistently produce the best results in the greatest percentage of the patients who come to them for treatment.* In the absence of outcome data, the quality of programs must be judged in terms of aspects of their functioning which are presumed to be related to good outcome. But that presumption may be incorrect. It is quite conceivable that a program could function with great efficiency and exhibit admirable characteristics, but fail to produce good results. Precisely this dilemma is embodied in the classical medical statement: "The operation was a success but the patient died."

The validity of this major reservation cannot be denied and, in the absence of outcome data, judgments as to quality must be viewed as presumptive rather than definitive. On the other hand, there is good reason why a preliminary assessment of quality ought to precede, rather than follow, studies of outcome. If such an assessment were to suggest problems, an outcome study would present difficulties in interpretation. The true potential of intervention can only be tested when a high quality of effort is involved. Therefore, as was concluded in the instance of drug abuse treatment programs, precise studies of outcome would ideally await the establishment of a logical and comprehensive system of treatment built of components of at least minimal quality. If this is not feasible, the results of outcome studies should be cautiously interpreted. They should be read not as indicating the ultimate capability of the treatment enterprise, but as a baseline reading on what is possible in the face of many difficulties.

The importance of such considerations was recognized in the Alaska survey. Its authors noted that "measurement of the successes or failures of a treatment with a patient needs to be related to the status of the patient when treatment is undertaken."[5] But the major finding of the survey was that the patient's initial status was not assessed; and, as was noted, "we cannot compare outcomes unless similar patients are compared."[6] Since it has already been shown (Chapter 4) that one of the most thorough-going needs in the Commonwealth is for compo-

* This statement assumes that only those methods of intervention are employed which are wholly ethical. It should not be read as indicating that good results justify the employment of any means which are necessary to achieve them.

nent II, which subserves precisely the function of evaluation, it is likely that outcome studies in Pennsylvania would face the same methodological problem.

There is some evidence that these difficulties have been recognized. An instrument designed for the assessment of drug dependent persons embodies a determination of the severity of the problem,[7] and is currently in use in the central intake program in Philadelphia. In the general area of mental health as well, there is presumptive evidence that programs of the same type, such as day programs, may deal with populations of patients having vastly different degrees of impairment, and that this must be taken into account in evaluation.[8] The Western Reserve Group, which performed the Alaska survey, suggest a means of doing this for alcoholism program patients which they call "staging." They feel that such a process would eventually improve the efficiency of treatment:

> *If the system requirements we have outlined can be accepted by agencies as standards of care, and if staging is used both as a change-measuring instrument and a way of comparing diagnosed alcoholics and treatment methods, perhaps we will be in a position to meaningfully compare treatment methods and choose the right patients for the proper treatment.*[9]

On the basis of these considerations, it was felt that some preliminary consideration of the quality of treatment being provided in the Commonwealth was in order. But as this was a subsidiary part of the survey, a modest means of quality assessment would have to be employed. The methodology utilized in the survey of drug abuse treatment programs[10] seemed reasonable for these purposes, and in addition would provide material for some comparisons between drug and alcohol treatment programs which might be of interest.

Methodology

Immediately after leaving each of the programs visited during the course of this survey, each member of the site-visiting team completed a post-site visit schedule. The schedule (Figure 1) permitted many of the practical details of the site visit to be recorded. It also embodied two rating scales. One was used to rate the degree of cooperation experienced by the site visitors, and the other to rate their global impressions of the program. Each scale was comprised of six points ranging from A through F.

Team members were instructed to think for a moment about their impressions of the program and then to choose that one of the six points which most closely approximated them. In-between grading (e.g. B− or C+) was not permitted, although many programs received such ratings as their consensus grades subsequently when the ratings

FIGURE 1

Post-Site Schedule

1. Name of Site:
2. Section Staff Present:
3. Hours at Site:
4. Major Events of the Day:
5. Persons Interviewed:
6. Ratings:
   - Extent of Cooperation toward Us — A B C D E F
   - Impression of Program — A B C D E F
7. Round-trip Miles ____________ Other Expenses ____________
8. Write Letters to:
9. Other:

of all observers for that program were mathematically averaged. The ratings of individual team members were separately recorded for each of the 80 programs. Subsequent to the completion of all site visits, the data were compiled and analyzed.

Of course, the power of such a simple methodology is not very great. The ratings are both global and impressionistic, and it is not entirely clear even in retrospect upon what factors they may have been based. They were not based on discrete criteria which were openly and systematically shared. The observations were made by differing combinations of observers with widely varying treatment and academic backgrounds. The total amount of time spent in the programs which were rated was almost certainly not a sufficient sample of that program's total experience. Moreover, the quality of a program's interventions is unlikely to be stable, but probably fluctuates over time. There is no guarantee that the survey team did not visit a particular program at a particularly low (or particularly high) point in its life history. Due to the long period of time over which the observations were made, there may have been considerable changes in the program, and hence these ratings cannot be considered current. The converse of these observations is that if serious attention is to be paid to the quality of treatment it must be monitored consistently and longitudinally.

Despite these very palpable limitations, the data to be presented are the only data extant on the quality of the entire group of alcoholism treatment programs in the Commonwealth of Pennsylvania. They represent consenus ratings by a professional research group which personally visited every program, and which neither operated programs of its own nor had any responsibility, fiscally or operationally, for the programs under review. Hence this was an independent and external assessment. Although its weaknesses are many, it also has its strengths. On balance, it may serve as an introduction to the problem of the quality of treatment for alcoholism in Pennsylvania.

Results

A total of seven separate team members were involved in site visits to alcoholism treatment programs in Pennsylvania. While this was perhaps a larger number than one might have wished, it was dictated by external circumstance rather than design and had, moreover, the advantage of broadening the perspective of the group as a whole. Collectively the group had experience in psychiatry, sociology, social work, epidemiology, anthropology, criminology, public health, and in the treatment of drug abuse and alcoholism, as well as in research generally. Three of the seven team members had participated in the field work of the drug abuse treatment study. No program was rated by only a single rater. Of all of the programs, 78.7% were rated by varying combinations of two team members, 10% by combinations of three, and 11.3% by combinations of four or more.

As was the case in the drug abuse survey, there was a very high degree of consistency among the raters. In terms of ratings on the cooperation experienced by the site-visiting teams, there was complete agreement in 71 out of the 80 programs visited. In the remaining nine programs the disagreement was within one letter grade in all cases. The more critical area of overall impression of treatment quality produced somewhat greater discrepancies. There was complete agreement in 54 of the 80 programs visited, or slightly over two thirds. In the remaining 26 programs the disagreement was within one letter grade in all but three instances. This suggests a very high degree of inter-rater agreement.

Ratings on the cooperation of programs were extremely high. Out of the total of all individual ratings, 83.8% were "A." This gratifying response was also noted in the drug abuse survey and, it is interesting to note, was commented upon by the authors of the Alaska survey: "Originally, a great amount of resistance was anticipated. Perhaps one of the biggest surprises was the enthusiastic welcome that was given at times to the study."[11] Once again the survey teams reported the regular expression of delight on the part of clinical personnel that their efforts were not going unnoticed. Those who take a dim view of research efforts in general should learn from this experience that they may at times generate good will rather than frustration. For the immediate purposes of this chapter it should be noted that the high degree of cooperation means that ratings of overall quality were *not* negatively influenced by a hostile reception of the site-visiting team; if anything there is likely to have been a halo effect, with ratings being given at a somewhat higher level than was merited in view of the cordiality of the team's reception.

TABLE 1

Consensus Ratings of 80 Pennsylvania Alcoholism Treatment Programs

Rating	No. Programs	% Programs
A	1	1.3
B	18	22.5
B–	2	2.5
C+	17	21.3
C	19	23.7
D+ and below	23	28.7
	80	100.0

It was all the more disquieting, therefore, to look at the results of the program ratings (Table 1). Only 21 of the 80 programs were rated as being of above average quality,* or only slightly more than a quarter of all programs (26.3%). These 21 programs contained only slightly more than a third (35.9%) of all of the patients in treatment. More than a quarter of all programs were consensually rated as being of below average quality. Phrased in the converse, the results indicate that almost three-quarters of all Pennsylvania treatment programs failed to achieve "good" quality, and that almost two-thirds of all patients in treatment were in these programs and hence were receiving less than a "good quality" of care.

* In the ensuing discussion the phrases "above average quality," "rating above C+," and "program(s) of 'good' quality" are considered identical. The word "good" is set off by quotation marks because, as noted above, in the absence of outcome data any judgments of quality are presumptive rather than definitive.

TABLE 2

Comparison of Consensus Ratings of 76 Pennsylvania Drug Abuse Treatment Programs and 80 Pennsylvania Alcoholism Treatment Programs.

Rating	% Drug Programs	% Alcohol Programs
Above Average	29.0	26.3
Average	39.5	45.0
Below Average	31.5	28.7
	100.0	100.0

X^2 = ns.

Although it is not the purpose of this report to compare drug and alcohol treatment programs, in this instance a comparison may be instructive. To make it more meaningful, consensus letter grades have been collapsed so that ratings from A to B- inclusive are subsumed in the Above Average ("Good") category; ratings of C+, C, and C− in the Average category; and all other ratings in the Below Average category. When this is done and the drug and alcohol programs are compared, the results are startlingly similar (Table 2). In fact, the differences do not achieve statistical significance.

Turning to the ratings of different kinds of programs, one finds that among the single-component programs those tending to receive the highest quality ratings were those in components III and IV, the "intensive" intervention and stabilization (halfway house) components. Consensus ratings above C+ were received by 55.5% of the component III and 40% of the component IV programs. However, the most striking finding among the single component programs was the relatively low consensus rating that component V programs received. Only 16.7% of these programs, which were the most frequent of all types of alcoholism treatment programs, were rated as being of "good" quality.

If all treatment programs are considered together, there is an apparent inverse relationship between the number of components in a program and the quality of the program (Table 3). While single-component programs and programs with a small number of components were rated as of "good" quality only about one quarter of the time, programs containing four or more components were rated as of "good" quality half of the time. It will be recalled from Chapter 4 that programs with four or more components have a branched schematic structure and are able to offer more than a single alternative treatment plan to their patients. Unfortunately, there are too few of these programs to allow for tests of the statistical significance of this finding, but the raw data are at least suggestive.

TABLE 3

Program Quality by Number of Components

No. Components	No. Above C+	% Above C+
1	14	24.6
2 - 3	5	27.8
4 - 5	2	50.0

Discussion

Even with due allowance being given to the unsophisticated nature of these data, these results are a matter for some concern. Most of the programs were not of "good" quality. Most patients in treatment were therefore not receiving a "good" quality of treatment. The most common type of program being utilized in the Commonwealth (component V), which has already been viewed on theoretical grounds as being the least satisfactory (Chapter 4), achieved only very low ratings. Conversely, the least common type of program, the multiple-component program with a branched structure, felt on theoretical grounds to be the most desirable, achieved high ratings. In a word, the overall picture was in some important respects exactly the opposite of what it optimally ought to have been. The most desirable programs, those with the highest ratings, were scarce; the least desirable programs, those with the lowest ratings, were common.

Further investigation of quality utilizing these data turned up some additional problems. For example, non-whites were under-represented in programs of "good" quality. Of all non-whites in treatment, 29.7% were in programs rated above C+, while 38.3% of all whites in treatment were in such programs. This difference is highly significant statistically, as was the case with respect to racial differences in drug abuse treatment programs. The data suggest that geographic factors are principally responsible for these differences. Of all blacks in the Commonwealth, 78.5% reside in the state's two urban areas, Philadelphia and Allegheny counties. Only seven of the 21 programs rated above C+ were to be found in these counties. Halfway houses and "intensive" treatment programs, those programs of the dominant single-component variety which were of the highest quality, were characteristically located outside of urban areas (14 of 19, or 73.7% in this survey). People tend to go to programs near where they live. But the fact that geographic factors weigh heavily in a consideration of treatment is itself a serious problem from a systems perspective. In medical terms, it is as if a man with a broken leg went to a psychiatric hospital for treatment because he happened to be living next door.

Rather than unduly taxing these limited data, one may simply say they suggest that additional attention be paid to the problem of quality of treatment, and ask whether they furnish any clues as to what may be done. In the study of drug abuse programs a number of factors could be found which might contribute to a high quality of treatment. This also turned out to be the case in the study of alcoholism treatment programs. In concluding this examination of the quality of treatment, some factors which may have contributed to these ratings are identified and discussed.

1. *Observer bias*. While this must be mentioned and is always a possibility, there is no *prima facie* reason to suppose that it accounts for the observed results. The complete revision of the taxonomy of

treatment programs, which occurred after all of the ratings had been made, militates against this factor. So does the greater number of observers and the many differing combinations of observers.

2. *Program structure* As noted above in Table 3, those programs which had a branched schematic structure (see also Chapter 4) appeared to be of higher quality than those which did not. These programs had a minimum of four components, one of which was evaluative (component II). Hence they could offer at least one alternative course of treatment to all of the patients who came within their purview. It may be speculated that the existence of these alternatives made a more careful evaluation of each patient imperative for such programs, and that the ensuing match between the patient's needs and the program's response to them resulted in a higher quality of treatment. Program personnel in such a structure would perforce have to think in terms of different treatments for different patients, and would avoid falling into the routinization and the conceptual ruts which sometimes characterized less sophisticated programs. The structure may also reflect a realization of the amount of effort required to effect a good result, and hence may be analogous to the factor of "total quantity of therapeutic effort" which was found to be of importance in the quality of drug abuse treatment programs. Of all of the factors identifiable in alcoholism treatment programs, this seemed to be the most significant at a subject level.

3. *Staff-patient ratio.* Those programs which were rated above C+ had one full-time staff member for every 9.1 patients, whereas those rated below C+ had one full-time staff member for every 14.9 patients, a rather considerable difference. It seems reasonable that a more favorable staff-patient ratio would result in a higher quality of intervention, particularly if it is accepted that a great deal of effort is required to produce a favorable result.

4. *Staffing pattern.* Programs rated as being of "good" quality made use of recovered alcoholics as personnel more than twice as frequently as did other programs. There was one such person for every 21.8 patients in the "good" programs as compared with one for every 48.5 patients in other programs. This parallels the findings in drug abuse treatment, where "good" programs also made more significant use of ex-addicts. In view of the empathy a former alcoholic may have for patients and his first-hand experience of the process of treatment, such a finding is not surprising.

5. *Program size.* In the drug abuse survey, program size was found to be inversely related to program quality: the larger the program, the less the quality. This seemed to be reversed in the present survey, where the "good" programs averaged 116.2 patients per program as opposed to 74.0 for other programs. However, since a high quality rating was associated with multiple components, a per-component figure is more instructive. Using this approach the discrepancy is narrowed: "good"

programs had 71.8 patients per component, while other programs had 51.4 patients per component. Not only are these differences less significant, but both figures are probably well within the "critical mass" which a program must exceed before quality begins to deteriorate. It should be remembered that in the drug survey a number of programs were encountered which had several hundred patients in a single setting. Hence the survey team continued to feel that program size was related to program quality, but that alcohol treatment programs have thus far avoided the problem by remaining within reasonable per-component limits. With mounting pressure to get an increased number of alcoholics into treatment, there will be a temptation to expand the size of existing programs rather than to create new ones. If this happens, the factor of program size could become operative with respect to diminution of quality. Such an eventuality should be guarded against.

6. *Management.* It was found that drug abuse treatment programs of "good" quality tended to have a higher complement of staff devoted to non-treatment activities, and the hypothesis was formulated that this might represent a superior quality of management which in turn permitted more adequate clinical care. The "good" alcoholism treatment programs failed to conform to this hypothesis, having *fewer* (1:46) such persons per patient than other programs (1:36). But the two sets of data may not be directly comparable. Since branched-chain programs with multiple components were correlated with higher quality, it might be argued that individual management personnel could be divided between the components and hence could be used more efficiently than in single component programs. When this is done in a rough manner it is found that "good" programs actually had 1.6 management personnel per component, whereas other programs had 1.4 management personnel per component. A more precise test would involve a far more complex design in which actual allocation of management personnel to components of multi-component programs, individual assessment of the quality of each component of multi-component programs, and individual counting of patients in each component would be undertaken at a minimum. It also should be remembered that the allocation of personnel is at best a crude indicator of the quality of management. The survey team continued to feel very strongly that the quality of a program's management was highly correlated with its overall quality.

No doubt the data on quality of treatment programs could be further teased to shed additional light on this very important problem. But data of such a limited degree of sophistication probably ought not to be bled white. Rather, they should be recognized as achieving, despite their shortcomings, three very important, if limited, goals. First, they suggest that the matter of quality of treatment requires attention. Second, they suggest that the interpretation of outcome evaluations may present difficulties. Improving the quality of existing components, supplementing them with new components, and forging the components into a comprehensive and rational treatment system should ideally be completed before outcome studies can provide us with a fair picture of what treatment at its best might accomplish in the field of problems related to alcohol. If this is not feasible, the results of outcome studies should be considered as baseline data, beyond which considerable improvement is possible.

Finally, the data suggest that it may be possible to identify certain general factors within programs which are correlated with a high quality of treatment. These factors may eventually prove to include the six listed above, or they may not; what the factors are is not as important as the probability that factors of this kind do exist and can be found. Once identified with certainty, they may prove to be readily transferable to all types of programs, and hence prove a boon to the entire treatment system. Clearly, more rigorous and extensive efforts to determine factors related to quality of treatment than those discussed in this chapter will be required to identify such factors with precision. But this study does indicate that such an effort may prove to be of value.

References

1. Adler, F., Moffett, A.D., Glaser, F.B., et al. *A Systems Approach to Drug Treatment.* Philadelphia: Dorrance & Co., 1975, Ch.13.
2. Glaser, F.B., Adler, F., Moffett, A.D., et al. The quality of treatment for drug abuse. *American Journal of Psychiatry, 131:* 598-601, May 1974.
3. Miller, S., Helmick, E., Berg, L., et al. Alcoholism: A state-wide program evaluation. *American Journal of Psychiatry: 131:* 210-14, February 1974, p.213.
4. *Ibid.*
5. *Ibid.,* p.211
6. *Ibid.,* p.213
7. Pittel, S.M., and Hofer, R. A systematic approach to drug abuse treatment referral. *Journal Psychedelic Drugs, 6:* 253-58, April-June 1974.
8. Glaser, F.B. The uses of the day program. *In:* Barten, H.H. and Bellak, L. (eds.). *Progress in Community Mental Health, vol.2,* New York: Grune & Stratton, 1972, pp.221-48.
9. Miller, *op.cit.,* p.213
10. Adler, et al., *op.cit.*
11. Miller, *op.cit.,* p.212.

Chapter 11

An Update of the Data

One of the few stable aspects of any mental health treatment system is its instability. Alcohol treatment in Pennsylvania is no exception. However, there are two kinds of instability. On the one hand, there is planned flexibility, such that programs grow and develop in response to the needs of the target population, needs that have been carefully gauged and examined. On the other hand, there is another type of instability, which is anathema to system development; it is a result of the random, directionless vicissitudes of individual programs. Unfortunately, it appears that the former is more the exception and the latter is more the rule in the current treatment enterprise.

In December of 1973, following the completion of the initial data collection, a follow-up letter was sent to every program visited. In order to encourage a high response rate, the letter contained a request for only three items of information—the number of alcohol patients, the number of full-time staff, and the number of part-time staff as of December 17, 1973. Almost 70% of the programs responded within two months; responses were received from the remaining programs via a second follow-up letter and phone calls.*

Given the fact that half of the programs were visited only six months prior to the mailing of the follow-up letter, the magnitude of change in the treatment system is all the more noteworthy.

* The follow-up data are based on 76 programs, since between the site visit and the follow-up letter, three programs were discontinued and one program failed to reply despite repeated phone calls and letters.

Between the initial data collection phase and follow-up, the number of patients in treatment increased by almost 20% from 6,805 to 7,978. Three-quarters of this increase took place in only two types of programs, combined detoxification/out-patient (I,V) programs, and comprehensive five-component programs. Proportionately, the greatest changes were found in detoxification (I) and combined halfway house/out-patient (IV,V) programs. Decreases occurred in only five program types, and in general they were not substantial.
substantial.

In contrast, during the same period, the full-time staff census declined, although the decrease was not as great as the increase in patients. Almost half the total decrease took place in a single type of program, intensive in-patient (III). Proportionately, the greatest decrease was found in combined detoxification/out-patient (I,V) programs, which lost over half of the staff. Out of 13 program types, only four had increases in staff size. This decline in full-time staff was not compensated for by part-time staff; all but three program types underwent a decrease in part-time staff, and the overall decrease in this category was 40%.

Given the increase in patients and the decrease in staff, the overall patient/staff ratio increased from nine to 12 patients per staff member. The most drastic changes took place in three program types—combined detoxification/out-patient (I,V), intensive in-patient/out-patient (III,V), and halfway house/out-patient (IV,V). Since all three have the common component of community based out-patient treatment, it is possible that system-wide changes in this component may account for the change although it is impossible to know for certain.

It would be misleading to assume that changes occurred uniformly within each program type. This was not the case, and in fact, the largest changes were often caused by one or two programs. An analysis within categories yielded the following findings:

... the substantial increase in both patients and staff of detoxification (I) facilities was entirely accounted for by the marked growth of one program.

... although there were no great changes in community based out-patient programs (V), six underwent patient decreases of 50% or more with little or no staff increase. In one such case, the staff was reduced from two to one.

... while there were few overall changes in halfway houses (IV), one program maintained a stable patient census but increased the staff by fourfold; another tripled the number of patients but had a decrease in staff from two to one.

... virtually all of the patient increase in combined detoxification/out-patient (I,V) programs took place in two facilities, one of which increased from 500 to 800 and the other from 200 to 630; at the same time, the staff declined from 21 to seven and 25 to eight, respectively.

... the single combined halfway house/out-patient program (IV,V) almost tripled its patient size, while the staff was decreased by one.

... one comprehensive five-component program doubled its patient census while the other lost almost one-quarter.

These findings indicate that, in most cases, changes in a given program type are the result of the vicissitudes of one or two individual facilities. This suggests that the overall increase in patients with a concurrent decrease in staff is not the product of planned flexibility to observed needs in the system or even developments within a specific type of treatment. Rather it appears to be random, sporadic, and without direction. There are a myriad explanations for drastic changes within programs, although it is impossible to know the specific situation in each case. For instance, increases in patients in a particular program could result from changes in law enforcement practices in the area in which the program is located, the closing of another program in the same community, inadequate screening of patients for appropriateness, or a sudden increase in the prevalence of alcoholism in the facility's area (a relatively unlikely cause of patient increase in a short period of time). The reasons for a sharp decrease in staff are just as diverse and difficult to predict. In fact, at least five programs have had a new director since the initial site visit, indicating an alarmingly rapid turnover of clinical leadership.

Not only do patients and staff come and go in an apparently erratic manner, but so do programs. Between the period of initial data collection and follow-up, three programs were discontinued. Since then, the research team has been made aware of the closing of another. The reasons are as disparate as the programs themselves, and reflect the haphazard condition of the current treatment enterprise. Three out of four programs were in urban areas and the other was in a small city. Beyond this, they have little in common. They were of various sizes and contained widely different treatment components. One closed for lack of funding; another appeared to have been the losing party in a local feud; still another was converted into an information and referral centre. Perhaps the most bizarre was a case in which the acting director of a program (a new director had not been hired after the former one left) was committed to a mental hospital. Shortly thereafter the owner of the property on which the facility was located, who was a recovered alcoholic and apparently quite active in the affairs of the program, was murdered. The program collapsed. Fortunately, most programs are not discontinued in such an abrupt manner. Nevertheless, these four cases illustrate the fact that the opening and closing of programs does not appear to be in response to changing needs of the target population but rather is random and unpredictable in most instances.

One-shot follow-ups of the type presented here cannot hope to convey a developmental view of the treatment enterprise in Pennsylvania. The best that can be hoped for currently is two snapshots at two points in time, and superficial ones at that. What is required is on-going, uniform monitoring of program activities on a system-wide basis. Traditionally, clinicians have balked at the requirements by all levels of government for the monthly completion of copious forms. They view it either as wasted time taken away from the treatment of patients or government eavesdropping for dubious purposes. Suspicion of "big brotherism" seems to be very much the temper of the times, and in many cases with good reason. However, the treatment enterprise can ill afford to reject out of hand valid attempts by state government to integrate and coordinate the treatment effort. The deleterious effects of a non-system are all too glaring to ignore steps taken toward the construction of a viable, comprehensive system.[1] One component of this process is the development of a uniform data collection system, which has recently been initiated by the single state agency. The advantages of such on-going monitoring are two-fold: it provides a source of continuous input for the purpose of planning, training, and research. Secondly, it promotes frequent communication between programs and coordinating body. If programs are treated as though they are units of a functioning system, they tend to view themselves in this light and eventually act accordingly.

In conclusion, we must emphasize the necessity for a permanent, on-going reciprocal relationship between treatment and research. This report offers only snapshot glances of the treatment enterprise at two points in time. If research, both original and applied, is to be developed to its full potential, it will have to be carried out at regular intervals. On the other hand, the programs will benefit by having readily available information on the treatment of alcoholism in the rest of the system. Further, the inclusion of all programs in a concrete, well-defined system is conducive to establishing frequent communication between programs in order to share ideas and problems, a relationship that cannot but help to improve the quality of treatment. Thus, rather than being viewed as yet another instance of intrusion on the part of "big brother," the reciprocal relationship between treatment and research has the potential for the development of truly innovative and effective responses to the problem of alcoholism.

References

1. Moffett, A.D., Greenberg, S.W., and Glaser, F.B. Non-programs in the management of drug and alcohol abuse. Presented at the National Drug Abuse Conference, Chicago, March 30-April 1, 1974.

Section Three

INTERVENTION EFFORTS OTHER THAN TREATMENT PROGRAMS

Chapter 12

Industrial Programs in Pennsylvania

The National Council on Alcoholism estimates that as many as 5% of the nation's workforce are alcoholic individuals and that almost another 5% are serious alcohol abusers.[1] This proportion is said to be increasing, but such estimates may reflect greater efficiency in the detection of alcoholics and a decreasing stigmatization of alcoholism rather than an absolute increase. Applying this estimate to the industrial workforce in Pennsylvania for 1972, the number of alcoholics employed in industry may have been as high as 75,000.

Alcohol abuse and alcoholism drain the nation's economy of an estimated $15 billion a year—$10 billion for lost work time in business, industry, government, and the military; $2 billion for health and welfare services provided to alcoholic persons and their families, property damage, and medical expenses; and $3 billion or more for overhead costs. It has been estimated that the annual cost of alcoholism to government, business, and industry in Pennsylvania alone is about $2 billion.[2]

As a response to this costly problem, a number of industrial corporations today have personnel policies consonant with the emerging view that alcohol-related problems can be dealt with effectively. In fact, it is estimated that the highest recovery rates may be found not in clinics and hospitals, but in offices and factories. By putting the body of knowledge about alcohol-related problems to work in company programs, industry is reporting recovery rates as high as 65 to 70%—higher than those for other major diseases and far higher for alcoholism than any imagined only a short time ago.[3] For example, Consolidated Edison in New York claims 60% success with employees, while DuPont in Delaware states that eight out of 10 of its problem drinkers are rehabilitated.

It is believed that the most important aspect of a successful recovery from alcoholism is the motivation to accept intervention, rather than the nature of the intervention itself. Industrial programs have one of the most effective motivational tools known—the desire of the employee to keep his job. Thus far, preliminary results have been heartening, as indicated by the recovery estimates of a number of programs.

Job-related alcohol programs were not a part of the original design of this study. For the most part, they do not conform to the definition of a treatment program which was utilized, in that they do not themselves provide definitive intervention. Moreover, there was the practical consideration that an exhaustive survey of employers in Pennsylvania to identify and then visit all such programs would have expanded the study effort beyond the realm of the possible. Nevertheless, the survey team felt increasingly throughout the course of the study that some attention must be paid to job-related programs, since the interaction of employment and alcohol-related problems continually thrust itself into their consideration and was obviously of considerable importance. (While it is not a major purpose of this study to draw comparisons, this did *not* happen during the course of the study of drug abuse treatment programs; although the interaction of work and drug abuse is no doubt important, it is clear that it is a different sort of interaction from that of work and alcohol abuse.)

As a compromise, the survey team elected to visit a number of job-related alcohol programs in the Philadelphia area, which were close to the team's base of operations and offered a variety of opportunities. Several of the programs are briefly described below. The most important result of this activity, however, was to suggest that in most instances places of employment had failed to concern themselves in any organized manner with alcohol-related problems, despite the fact that such problems were universally recognized to be widespread and critical. An absence of leadership and knowledge was most frequently cited in explaining this lack of activity.

Accordingly, in a subsequent portion of the chapter, a possible model for the management of alcohol-related problems in the job situation will be presented. The model is designed primarily to assist in the establishment of an actual treatment program. It is felt that this constitutes the minimum program which every place of employment ought to establish. Many work situations will wish to go beyond this model and to consider the provision of actual treatment services within the context of the job. This has already happened in some larger companies, both with respect to alcoholism and health problems generally. Smaller companies seem to have a particular problem in mounting such programs, even though the need is no less great, and perhaps should consider the formation of inter-company *consortia.* The so-called HMO's (health maintenance organizations) to be widely established under new federal legislation may be considered a model for this approach.

In any case, it is clear that a great deal more attention needs to be paid to job-related problems with alcohol. It is mainly to emphasize this point that the survey now departs from its usual format to present material based more upon theory than upon actual field research. There are many problems yet to be resolved. For example, although a management-based model has been evolved and will be presented below, labor has argued forcibly that, in view of its traditional concern for health matters, such systems should find their anchor in that sphere, with (for example) the key figure being the shop steward rather than the supervisor. There are merits on both sides of the argument, and it is obvious that the solutions to these and other problems will have to be worked out between labor and management in the usual manner. Fortunately, all agree that more needs to be done. The chapter therefore concludes with a strong suggestion that further effort in this area become a high priority item for the future.

Industrial Alcoholism Programs in the Philadelphia Area

The research team visited several programs in the Philadelphia area which provide alcoholism services for troubled employees. Calls and letters were directed to other industries in order to request a site visit, but no response was ever received.

In one large company, the medical director heads the entire program and assists in counseling. In addition, the company employs the services of an Alcoholics Anonymous counselor, who works three days a week. In addition to counseling, he renders weekly educational lectures to management and supervisors. The program is geared to train supervisors to recognize (without making a medical diagnosis) problem drinkers in their department. When an employee is suspected of having a drinking problem he is immediately referred to the medical department for follow-up; occasionally a patient is hospitalized in an alcoholic rehabilitation hospital. All patients are encouraged to affiliate with AA and attend meetings within the plant. An AA sponsor, who is also a company employee, is provided for each patient. Wives of alcoholics are also interviewed periodically and are encouraged to join Al-Anon. It was reported to the research team that labor unions have been most cooperative and supportive of the program.

Another large company has an active program for alcoholic employees that is supported by a formalized, written company policy, entitled "The Misuse of Alcohol." Because of familiarity with an employee's attendance record, job performance, and appearance on the job, the supervisor is in the best position to recognize that an employee may have a drinking problem. The supervisor is urged neither to ignore a suspected drinker in his unit, nor to cover up for him. The sooner the supervisor acts, the better for all concerned.

When an employee's performance, productivity, or attendance pattern is altered as a result of excessive drinking, the personnel department is consulted and an immediate referral is made to the medical office. Following the medical examination, the employee's supervisor and the personnel representative of his department, in consultation with the doctor, will make a decision either to actively participate in the rehabilitation of the employee or to advise the employee to assume the responsibility for seeking treatment. If rehabilitation is undertaken, the medical consultant assists the supervisor and personnel representative in developing and carrying out a program suited to the individual. If the latter measure is deemed advisable, the employee is guided to an appropriate source of treatment in the community.

In reaching a decision, the basic premise is that the company cannot retain an habitual non-performer on its rolls. However, it may be desirable to attempt to correct the problem by further measures, including:

1. demotion to less demanding work;
2. suspension;
3. leave of absence.

The company stresses the importance that the supervisor, personnel representative, and doctor closely follow the employee's progress and express continual interest and concern. Rehabilitation measures are modified promptly whenever indicated. Follow-up is pursued whether the employee continues to work, is institutionalized, or is suspended.

For two other companies it appeared that AA was almost solely responsible for providing care to employees with drinking problems. The paucity of company resources available for the worker plagued by problem drinking is perhaps attributable to the newness of the alcohol programs in both companies. There are several other possible reasons for this marked tendency. One may be that Alcoholics Anonymous has been recognized as a relatively successful program for over 30 years. Another reason may have to do with economics. It is obviously much less expensive to utilize the services of an already existing organization than for the company to take the responsibility of initiating its own program. However, in view of the impressive results achieved by a number of industrial programs, it would be desirable for large companies eventually to establish their own programs, while continuing to utilize Alcoholics Anonymous as a valuable community resource.

Program Design

Alcoholism programs are generally based on the premise that alcoholism is a tractable problem from which, with proper assistance, the individual can be extricated and be retained as a satisfactory employee. The following policy implementation plan has been suggested[5] to help the supervisor in dealing with problem drinkers on his staff.

1. Deal with the employee in a forthright manner within established administrative procedures.
2. Make no attempt to hide the diagnosis of problem drinking.
3. The problem drinker, once identified, will be encouraged to secure medical or other professional help.
4. The employee will receive disciplinary action only if treatment is proven unsuccessful or if he has refused to seek help.
5. Disciplinary action will involve temporary lay-off, which could lead to termination of employment. If the employee is adversely affected by his alcohol-associated behavior, his suspension may be immediate.

As can be seen, the principal policy objective is to retain employees who are developing a drinking problem by encouraging them to accept treatment before they become unemployable. Discharge is not the best answer to a costly personnel problem. A much more effective method is a forthright, treatment-oriented approach which allows the employee to face his illness by guiding him to experienced lay and professional groups for treatment. As such, the proposed industrial alcoholism control program is preventive in the sense that its primary objective is to avoid further progression of the disease as soon as possible after detection.

The Supervisor—a Key Person

The immediate supervisor of the employee is the key to the success of the program. On the one hand, it is the supervisor who is directly aware of the absenteeism, the errors, the personality problems, the deteriorating job performance, and the developing problem with alcohol. But on the other hand, the supervisor has much to gain in retaining a trained employee. Because of his position as an intermediary between labor and management, he may be the one person who is best situated to motivate the employee to stop drinking and seek help; when confronted by his supervisor it is difficult for the employee to ignore the effects of his problem on job performance and the possibility that his job is in jeopardy.

Understanding that the diagnosis of alcoholism is to be left for professionally-trained personnel, the supervisor has three basic responsibilities:

1. Identifying as early as possible a job-involved problem, possibly related to drinking;

2. Discussing the problem in an interview with the employee to suggest ways of correcting the problem;
3. Making a decisive plan of action with the employee, supported by a superior officer or a representative of the personnel department.

Although not an expert, the supervisor should know how to spot early symptoms through deteriorating job performance; how to refer the employee to the proper source of help; and what resources are available to assist him in handling the problem employee.

The principal factors that will determine action to be taken in dealing with an employee with a drinking problem are:

1. The nature and seriousness of the work-involved problem;
2. The type of work involved and the morale problem of the work group affected;
3. The desire of the employee to work on his problem as manifested by the steps he takes to secure help;
4. The progress of the treatment.

Once these factors have been taken into account and it is determined that alcohol may be the basis of the problem, the supervisor takes the following steps:

1. *The Initial Interview.* This should consist of a frank and open discussion between the employee and his immediate supervisor, during which the employee is appraised of the situation as his supervisor views it. This appraisal should be based on previously *recorded facts* relative to the employee's job performance, absenteeism, alteration of behavior, appearance and physical condition, and general attitudes. Following this, a plan of action is discussed and the employee is encouraged to follow it.

Whether the employee admits or denies his problem, the initial consultation is designed to leave him with the knowledge that something is interfering with his job performance and that he is expected to take the responsibility in alleviating the situation. He should have the impression that his employer is in full sympathy with his problem and will cooperate within reason when the employee takes positive steps to effect an improvement.

The employee is urged to make an immediate appointment to discuss his problem with a counselor. He is asked to report back to his supervisor within one week on his plan of getting help. The employee's voluntary action at this stage permits the easiest solution of the problem and assures *confidentiality.*

Further, this interview serves to apprise the employee of his endangered position and to make it clear that the job-related problem is primarily his, that the outcome will be of his own determination, and that his department's understanding and assistance will be in direct proportion to his own initiative and progress toward a satisfactory solution. A written report of this meeting will be made by the supervisor, with the employee's knowledge.

A medical rehabilitation office will be notified of this referral both by telephone and memorandum. If an employee fails to contact the medical rehabilitation office, it will notify the employee's supervisor.

2. *A Second Interview with the Problem Employee.* If the employee denies that alcohol is a problem or if the voluntary effort described fails to produce results, further action by the supervisor is necessary. A second interview is the next step, the purpose of which is to force the problem into the open. It should include the supervisor, a division head, a representative from personnel, and if possible, the assigned rehabilitation counselor. At this time, the employee is expected to express honestly his attitudes concerning both the problem and the recommendations that have been made to deal with it.

It should be made clear to the employee that the problem is of sufficient severity to require him to go to his own family physician or to a designated physician for an examination in order to determine, if possible, whether a factor other than alcohol is causing the problem. The employee will be urged to accept such referral, and upon acceptance, the employee's supervisor will notify, both by telephone and in writing, the medical rehabilitation office. A written record will be kept of all meetings and their outcome, with the employee's knowledge.

3. *Implementation of a Rehabilitation Program.* When the recommendations from the medical office have been received, the employee is again interviewed by the supervisor, division head, personnel representative, and rehabilitation counselor. Depending on the recommendations made, a time schedule will be set up which the employee will be urged to accept.

If institutional or other treatment is indicated, the employee will be granted leave within the limits of his accumulated sick and vacation leave. Additional leave of absence without pay may be granted by the employing agency, not to exceed a period of six months. If at the end of this leave period an extension of time for treatment is requested, the employer may grant a further period of time off without pay, again not to exceed six months.

If the situation does not warrant institutional treatment, a reasonable period of time will be agreed upon during which the worker is expected to make substantial inroads in handling the problem. If the employee refuses treatment, discipline will commence the very next time drinking interferes with the employee's job performance.

A written record will be kept of the meeting and an action recommended in this step, with the knowledge of the employee.

4. *Disciplinary Action, if Needed.* This step is necessary only if there is a continuation of a problem with alcohol or if medical consultation is refused. The recurrence of poor or faulty work will be frankly discussed with the employee, and a disciplinary suspension without pay, not to exceed five working days, should be arranged by the employer, to take

effect immediately. The employee will once again be apprised of the department's willingness to assist him in getting appropriate help. He shall be told that if his illness continues to interfere with his work he will face further disciplinary action which will culminate in termination of employment.

5. *Continued Deterioration of Job Performance.* An unwillingness on the part of the alcoholic employee to improve his condition will lead to termination of employment following the second or third suspension, depending on the severity with which his drinking affects job performance.

A summary report with all action taken and the subsequent outcome will be prepared for the records of the employer.

Consultation Service

The office of the rehabilitation service will be available for consultation to supervisors and personnel officers on matters regarding the alcoholism program and problem employees. The staff of this office should not work directly with any employee who has a drinking problem. Rather, arrangements may be made for a description or presentation of the problem drinker to any group of interested supervisors or other management personnel.

TABLE 1
(Reference 4)

Signs of Developing Alcoholism

1. Leaving post temporarily
2. Drinking at lunch time
3. Red or bleary eyes
4. Mood changes after lunch
5. Lower quality of work
6. Absenteeism: day or half day
7. More unusual excuses of absence
8. Loud talking
9. Longer lunch periods
10. Hand tremors
11. Lower quantity of work
12. Hangovers on job
13. Drinking during working hours
14. Avoiding boss or associates
15. Flushed face
16. Less even, more spasmodic work pace
17. Increase in real minor illnesses

TABLE 2
(Reference 4)

Frequency of Signs of Developing Alcoholism

TYPE	SIGN
1. Noticeable early, frequently thereafter.	Absenteeism: half day or day Leaving post temporarily More unusual excuses for absences Lower quality of work Mood changes after lunch Red or bleary eyes
2. Noticeable later, but frequently thereafter,	Less even, more spasmodic work pace Lower quantity of work Hangovers on job
3. Noticeable fairly early, but infrequently thereafter	Loud talking Drinking during lunch time Longer lunch periods Hand tremors
4. Noticeable late and infrequently thereafter.	Drinking during working hours Avoiding boss or associates Flushed face Increase in real minor illnesses

Guide for Supervisors for Identifying the Alcoholic Employee

Studies have indicated that supervisors are in a favorable position to observe many of the early and recurring signs of developing alcoholism among their employees. The signs that are most likely to be noticed by supervisors are primarily behavioral and tend to be related to job performance.[4]

Table 1 lists 17 signs most often checked by supervisors as being among the first five signs of alcoholism, while Table 2 lists the frequency of the signs of developing alcoholism. While such indicators are somewhat imprecise and tend to vary among individuals, they have been shown to be quite helpful as an aid in the early detection of problem drinking.

Leadership Initiatives from Governmental and Private Sectors

The first Labor and Management Alcoholism Conference was held in 1964 at the Penn Harris Hotel in Harrisburg and was sponsored by the first Governor's Advisory Council on Alcoholism. It was the unanimous opinion of all participants that future progress in the management of alcoholism in industry depends upon the recognition and acceptance by both labor and management that alcoholism is a chronic illness and those affected with this disorder should be treated. It was determined there must be a willingness on the part of the company and union to provide for the patient with alcoholism the same protection and financial security given to other employees having an acute or chronic illness.

During the past several years, the Commonwealth has taken specific steps to recognize and attempt to alleviate the problem of alcoholism in industry. These activities climaxed with a conference for labor and management on September 10, 1974, sponsored by the Governor's Council on Drug and Alcohol Abuse. Over 300 labor-management representatives and drug and alcohol specialists throughout the state attended the conference.

Ten years ago there were very few companies with a program for alcoholism. The policy at the time was to discharge the offending employee without even an offer to help with the employee's problem. Today, 15 companies throughout the Commonwealth have policies which offer the employee an opportunity to seek treatment while protecting his job. A score of other companies have programs based on job performance ratings for helping the employee suffering from alcoholism.

It has become increasingly important to assist management and the labor unions in developing a better understanding of this illness. To accomplish this, another recommendation from the first conference was put into operation. Many Alcohol Education Courses were conducted for labor union personnel and more recently for supervisory personnel at the management level. The important role of the community voluntary and public agencies in promoting and directing education programs in providing treatment and rehabilitation facilities for the alcoholic was considered as essential then as now.

The Governor's Council on Drug and Alcohol Abuse, in one of its earlier meetings, recognized the significance of retaining and implementing the Occupational Alcoholism Program, which was already in existence at the time of the Council's organization. Three staff members are employed full-time to work with labor and management to conduct courses on alcohol education, to assist with policy development, and to train key personnel within industry and the local Drug and Alcohol Councils to further develop programs on alcohol problems within the industrial community.

Conclusions

The employment situation provides an excellent opportunity for the early detection of and intervention in alcoholism. When the employee begins to be less efficient in his job because of his alcohol problem, the employer is in a unique position to intervene with knowledgeable and effective assistance. If, at the earliest signs of job performance impairment, the employer would take the initiative, the alcoholic would be forced to confront his problem much earlier than otherwise, and could therefore deal with it from a position of relative strength and support.

For these reasons, the research team recommends that the Governor's Council on Drug and Alcohol Abuse formulate plans for the funding of pilot alcohol programs in government, business, and industry. Ideally, these programs should be closely coordinated with all other available community resources. The guidelines for the state program should come from those government, business, and industrial programs which are already operating successfully throughout the country. The state program could, in turn, serve as a model for similar programs throughout Pennsylvania in both the public and private sectors. The primary aims of such a program should be prevention, early detection, and treatment of alcoholism among employed alcoholics in all walks of life.

References

1. Prevalence of alcoholism among employees. Industrial Services Department, National Council on Alcoholism, March 19, 1968. (unpublished report)

2. Barrett, M. *The Pennsylvania state alcohol abuse and alcoholism plan for 1971-1972* Harrisburg: Commonwealth of Pennsylvania, 1972.

3. Business Copes with Alcoholics. *Business Week,* October 26, 1968; also, H. Maurer. The beginning of wisdom about alcoholism. *Fortune,* May 1968.

4. Plaut, T.F.A. *Alcohol problems: A report to the nation.* New York: Oxford University Press, 1967.

5. Maxwell, M. Early identification of problem drinkers in industry. *Journal of Studies on Alcohol* Vol. *21:* 655-678, 1968.

Chapter 13

Alcoholics Anonymous

In the past 35 years, Alcoholics Anonymous has become one of the best known, and in some ways, one of the most enigmatic organizations for the treatment of alcoholism. Termed a fellowship by its members, AA is comprised of semi-autonomous groups of alcoholics whose sole mission is to keep sober. The goal of AA members is to help fellow alcoholics achieve sobriety and, in doing so, maintain their own sobriety. The organization has vigorously avoided involvement with other mental health or social problems. As one of its guidelines states: "Each group has but one purpose—to carry its message to the alcoholic who still suffers."

From a therapeutic perspective, Alcoholics Anonymous is a fascinating organization. It is lauded as one of the most successful ways of dealing with alcoholism, with over 17,000 groups throughout the world having a membership exceeding 575,000 in 1972.[1] Yet it does not make use of the professionals usually involved in the treatment of alcoholism. In addition, it operates solely on the contributions of its members and flatly refuses offerings from private individuals or government. Further, while attempts have been made, AA has remained essentially impervious to thorough and detailed evaluations of its effectiveness.[2] In order to gain some understanding of this unique organization, let us look at its development, its program, and its importance in the treatment of alcoholism in Pennsylvania.

Development

The founder of Alcoholics Anonymous, Bill W. was pronounced a hopeless alcoholic in 1934 while undergoing one of dozens of detoxifications at the Towns Hospital in New York. Following this gloomy prognostication by Dr. William Silkworth, he continued to drink heavily on and off for months. By coincidence he happened to renew his acquaintanceship with Eddy T., an old school friend and drinking partner. This meeting was to form the germ from which AA grew.

Ebby T., also a chronic alcoholic, had recently joined the Oxford Group Movement, perhaps the single most important historical influence on AA. Known originally as the First Century Christian Fellowship, and currently as Moral Re-Armament, the organization was founded in 1921 by Dr. Frank Buchman, a Lutheran clergyman and a native of Pennsylvania. It is essentially an evangelistic organization, devoted to combating the "oncoming forces of materialism." Its guiding principles are threefold: the world of men is sinful and in need of spiritual regeneration; this regeneration can be accomplished only through changing individuals; and direct guidance from God is available to those who surrender their will to Him. Since both personal and social problems are believed to be grounded in the individual, the goal of the Oxford Group Movement is to change lives.[4]

To this end, Buchman and his followers devised a detailed course of action. Essentially, it involved five steps known as the "five Cs"—confidence, confession, conviction, conversion, and continuance.[5] In order to achieve this life-changing, members would gather in private homes or hotels for what were known as "house parties." Buchman believed that real change could only come about in a public situation, and therefore all significant events in the Oxford Group Movement took place in gatherings of 10 or more. Perhaps the most important mechanism for change is public confession. At each meeting, several members gave detailed accounts of their sinful way of life, consequent unhappiness, and subsequent surrender to God. The intention was to show others that all men are sinful, but spiritual rebirth was available to everyone simply by following the Group's precepts.[6] Membership to the Oxford Group was open to anyone who had the desire to make a fundamental change in his life. One of their slogans was "you can't join; you can't resign; you are either in or out by the quality of life you lead." However, loyalty and deference were supposed to be extended toward experienced life changers, and novices usually had sponsors.[7]

While the Oxford Group did not have a specific program for alcoholics, Buchman and his disciples felt that alcoholism could be cured by assiduously following their program. (However, they later became discouraged with their failure to change the lives of alcoholics and believed that perhaps they presented special problems that the Group was not prepared to handle.) When Eddy T. first spoke with Bill W. he presented him with the following tenets:

> *You admit you are licked; you get honest with yourself; you talk it out with somebody else; you make restitution to the people you have harmed; and you pray to whatever God you think there is, even as an experiment.*[8]

With some minor modification, this statement came to be the nucleus around which AA was formed. In addition, the practice of one alcoholic sharing his strengths and weaknesses with another received its inception at these early meetings with Ebby T. and Bill W., although the latter did not realize their significance immediately.

Several months after his initial conversation with Ebby T., Bill W. again underwent a "drying-out" period at the Towns Hospital. He felt as if he had hit an emotional nadir. However, one night he experienced a spiritual awakening which convinced him that the only road to sanity was via helping other alcoholics. Shortly thereafter, he became associated with the Oxford Group. However, his efforts were largely unsuccessful. There were several reasons for the lack of efficacy of the Oxford Group approach: it was not specifically directed toward alcoholics; there was an over-emphasis on the four moral absolutes of purity, unselfishness, love, and honesty; and it was unsympathetic to Bill W.'s insistence on anonymity, which he felt was required on account of the shame attached to an admission of alcoholism.[9]

In 1935, on a business trip to Akron, Bill W. sought out a fellow alcoholic because he felt the return of his old urge to drink. He encountered Dr. Bob, a local surgeon with a long-standing drinking problem. Rather than preaching the moral absolutes of the Oxford group, Bill simply related to Dr. Bob his experiences as a life-long drinker and his road back to health. In addition, he employed for the first time what later became AA's working definition of alcoholism, an allergy plus an obsession. Simply stated, the alcoholics are physically allergic to alcohol and therefore have an allergic reaction whenever they drink; in addition there is a psychological obsession with drinking.[10]

As a direct result of this interaction, Dr. Bob took his last drink, which marked the official birth of AA. The concepts and techniques used by Bill W. in the original encounter became the basis for the AA approach. During the next few years, its message and procedure were carried to several large cities, including Philadelphia. By the end of 1937, Bill W. and Dr. Bob counted 40 alcoholics who had become sober as a result of the AA program.

Philadelphia was perhaps more important for the growth and

development of AA than any other city, except Akron and New York. It was through the interest of three Philadelphia physicians, Drs. A. Wiese Hammer, C. Dudley Saul, and John F. Stouffer, that an AA chapter was initiated in this city in 1940. Through their efforts, hospital care for alcoholics was improved and a detoxification clinic was started. In addition, a friend of Dr. Hammer's happened to be one of the editors of the *Saturday Evening Post.* This coincidence resulted in a feature story on AA which appeared in the *Post* in 1941. Following its appearance, thousands wrote in asking for help. By the end of 1941, membership had increased from 2,000 in 1940 to 8,000 and had spread into Canada and other foreign countries. Thus, Philadelphia figures centrally, if somewhat indirectly, in the history of AA.

During this period, there was a second event which had a profound effect on its development. Because of their dire need for funds, Dr. Bob and Bill W. approached John D. Rockefeller, Jr., in 1937. However, Rockefeller immediately recognized that the donation of a large sum of money would violate one of AA's most fundamental organizational principles—to be self-supporting—and might lend it an air of professionalism. On this basis, he agreed to donate $5,000 to allay its immediate needs and advised Dr. Bob and Bill W. that the remainder would have to come from the organization itself, as stated in Tradition 7. This action set AA firmly on the path which it has followed ever since.

The AA Program

There can be no discussion of the AA program without reference to the Twelve Steps and Twelve Traditions. The former represents its ideology, while the latter its formal organizational structure.

Twelve Suggested Steps of Alcoholics Anonymous

1. We admitted we were powerless over alcohol—that our lives had become unmanageable.
2. Came to believe that a Power greater than ourselves could restore us to sanity.
3. Made a decision to turn our will and our lives over to the care of God as we understood Him.
4. Made a searching and fearless moral inventory of ourselves.
5. Admitted to God, to ourselves, and to another human being the exact nature of our wrongs.
6. Were entirely ready to have God remove all these defects of character.
7. Humbly asked Him to remove our shortcomings.
8. Made a list of all persons we had harmed, and became willing to make amends to them all.
9. Made direct amends to such people wherever possible, except when to do so would injure them or others.

10. Continued to take personal inventory and when we were wrong promptly admitted it.
11. Sought through prayer and meditation to improve our conscious contact with God as we understood Him, praying only for knowledge of His will for us and the power to carry that out.
12. Having had a spiritual awakening as the result of these steps, we tried to carry this message to alcoholics and to practise these principles in all our affairs.

As can be seen, the influence of the Oxford Group is pervasive. The major foci of this group are all present—surrendering the will to a higher Power, sharing weaknesses with others, making amends to people who have been harmed, undergoing spiritual rejuvenation, and carrying the message to others. This last, Step 12, is central to the AA program. Making 12th Step calls is considered essential to maintaining sobriety, and the norms of the organization strongly support this activity. Whenever an alcoholic calls an AA office asking for help, the members (usually a team of two) are expected to respond immediately by calling on the alcoholic.[11] While new members may not be asked to do 12th Step work, those who have been in the fellowship for some time generally define this as an integral part of their role. It is considered to be one of the most important ways of carrying the message to alcoholics.

The Twelve Traditions of Alcoholics Anonymous

1. Our common welfare should come first; personal recovery depends upon AA unity.
2. For our group purpose there is but one ultimate authority—a loving God as He may express Himself in our group conscience. Our leaders are but trusted servants; they do not govern.
3. The only requirement for AA membership is a desire to stop drinking.
4. Each group should be autonomous except in matters affecting other groups of AA as a whole.
5. Each group has but one primary purpose—to carry its message to the alcoholic who still suffers.
6. An AA group ought never endorse, finance, or lend the AA name to any related facility or outside enterprise lest problems of money, property, and prestige divert us from our primary purpose.
7. Every AA group ought to be fully self-supporting, declining outside contributions.
8. Alcoholics Anonymous should remain forever non-professional, but our service centres may employ special workers.
9. AA, as such, ought never be organized; but we may create service boards or committees directly responsible to those they serve.
10. Alcoholics Anonymous has no opinion on outside issues, hence the AA name ought never be drawn into public controversy.

11. Our public relations policy is based on attraction rather than promotion; we need always maintain personal anonymity at the level of press, radio, and films.
12. Anonymity is the spiritual foundation of our traditions, ever reminding us to place principles before personalities.

The Twelve Traditions delineate the organizational structure. In effect, they are the organizational means of obtaining the ideological ends outlined in the Steps. Contrary to the latter, the Traditions represent a sharp break from the structure of the Oxford Group in that they strongly recommend limiting their activities exclusively to helping the alcoholic, rejecting contributions, avoiding controversy, and maintaining anonymity.

Components of the Program

Disease Concept. One of the turning points in Bill W.'s attainment of sobriety was his re-definition of alcoholism as a disease—an allergy plus an obsession. This concept is central to the AA ideology. In essence, alcoholism is redefined from a moral or personality weakness to a disease, like cancer or diabetes. Individuals are thereby relieved of responsibility for the etiology of the ailment since they cannot be blamed for contracting a disease. They are then free to concentrate their efforts on combating the symptoms. In addition, they are no longer constrained to regard themselves as a social outcast.[12] It is felt that this emphasis on symptoms rather than causes is one of AA's major strengths.[13,14] However, one of the corollaries is an insistence on abstinence. Just as a person who is allergic to strawberries would avoid eating them at all costs, an alcoholic must abstain from alcohol. This prescription is of such importance that it is the first of the Twelve Steps; it is necessary to master it before continuing with the rest of the program. Significantly, the only membership requirement is the desire to stop drinking. If individuals continue to drink with no indication they intend to stop, for all intents and purposes, they are no longer members.

Spirituality. One of the principles of the AA program is the necessity of having a spiritual awakening as a requisite to sobriety. In fact, AA would probably assert that spirituality is not simply a component of the program but rather it *is* the program. Essentially, the spiritual message is that individuals must transcend themselves and surrender their will to a Higher Power. Most people define this Power as God in the Judaeo-Christian sense, but it is emphasized that alcoholics are free to define this concept in their own way, perhaps even through the deification of the AA group itself. Alcoholics Anonymous holds that the common characteristic of all alcoholics is their tendency to get drunk on their own ego, their inability to look outside of themselves. Therefore, the only way to sobriety is to surrender their will to an external force. This ideology is pervasive throughout the Twelve Steps and in several of the Traditions. The substance of the spiritual message can be traced directly, with minor modifications, to the Oxford Group Movement and is at least partially an attempt to draw strength from Bill W.'s religious experience, which was vital to the inception of AA.

While AA stresses the importance of a spiritual awakening, it fervently denies that it is either an organized religion or an ideology. Rather it is a fellowship whose sole purpose is to help the alcoholic to stop drinking. However, several students of the organization have commented on its cult-like features. For example, a characteristic common to all religions is the prescription to transcend the self and to draw strength from an external power. The weaknesses and transience of the individual are usually a focal point. Secondly, most religions are concerned with carrying the new way of life (i.e. sobriety through spirituality) to those who are not yet converted.[15] Alcoholics Anonymous attempts to accomplish this goal via the 12th Step call, referred to above. While it does not recruit members, once the alcoholics make the initial contact, every effort is made to incorporate them into the group. Lastly, religions that were started by a charismatic leader form a cult around this person after his death in an attempt to maintain the group's initial fervor. In the case of AA, Bill W. and to a lesser extent, Dr. Bob, fulfill this function. Their comments on each of the Twelve Traditions, along with those of the original members, are collected in a volume known as the *Big Book,* the AA equivalent of Holy Writ. Their words are regarded as inspired and in some types of meetings, this book and other official AA publications are used in a way that is strikingly similar to a religious service. In addition, the houses in Akron and New York in which the first meetings were held have been virtually enshrined. Thus, while AA is not manifestly religious, there does seem to be a religious quality in both its form and substance. Even though members would vehemently deny this, perhaps this quality is one of their strengths in terms of extending their message to alcoholics, and retaining them in the group.

Anonymity. A direct corollary of the spiritual component of AA is the importance of anonymity, both in a personal and an organizational sense. As Tradition 12 states, "Anonymity is the spiritual foundation of our traditions, ever reminding us to place principles before personalities." During all AA functions, members address each other by first names only or first names and last initials. On the level of the organization, there is also anonymity in that AA will not endorse other groups, is completely self-supporting, will not become involved in public controversy, and does not engage in public relations. The rationale for this is fourfold. First, it is a way of protecting members from the stigma of being publically identified as alcoholics. Secondly, within AA, alcoholism is the only significant characteristic of the individual; all else is unimportant. Thirdly, it is felt that most alcoholics have spent their lives trying to inflate their own egos, usually without success. In effect, the alcoholic gets drunk on his ego. This point was made clear to us when we attended a meeting of a Philadelphia chapter of AA. At the beginning of the meeting, the leader for that evening announced that he had received a request from a large alcoholism treatment facility to have AA members counsel patients on a voluntary one-to-one basis. One of the members vociferously objected to the request on the grounds that the help offered by AA is based on group meetings, that in fact, all significant activities (other than 12th Step calls) take place in a group context. Finally, the founders of AA were aware from the beginning of the ill-fate suffered by an earlier movement to help alcoholics. The Washingtonian Society, founded in Baltimore over a century ago, was similar in many respects to AA. It was a self-help group comprised solely of alcoholics. At its zenith, its membership exceeded 500,000. However, the organization permitted itself to be used by politicians and reformers to further such causes as abolition and temperance. The members became so involved in political activity that the original momentum for helping alcoholics was lost, and the movement finally collapsed. As stated above, the only way to sobriety, according to AA, is to transcend the self and surrender the will to a Higher Power. Therefore, anonymity, both individually and organizationally, is intrinsic to this goal.

Meetings. AA meetings are the core of its being. They are the vehicle for extending such messages as the disease concept, spiritual awakening, the importance of anonymity, and most importantly, the Twelve Steps and Twelve Traditions. Without them, the fellowship would not be viable. While the only criterion for membership is the desire to stop drinking and members are not obligated to attend a certain number of meetings, in order to derive the benefits of the fellowship it is necessary to attend meetings regularly. For the most part, it is here that the message is presented.

There are four types of meetings—open, closed, step, and beginners. At the open meetings, the general public is invited to attend. Basically, the open meeting consists of the presentations of several alcoholics, usually two, who recount their story of their life as an alcoholic and their recovery through the AA program. Afterwards, the meeting breaks up into small informal discussion groups where alcoholism and AA are discussed over coffee. This is sometimes known as "coffee therapy." At closed meetings, to which only alcoholics are invited, the members submit questions to the discussion leader for that week. He offers suggestions and then opens up the issue to general discussion. Step meetings consist of the discussion of a single step, each member offering his own experience in dealing with that step. All meetings are ended by the passing of the collection basket, the recitation of the Lord's Prayer, and adjournment to informal groups. Finally, the beginner's meeting is held prior to the regular meeting by a long-term member in order to acquaint newcomers with the AA program.[16]

In addition to the manifest function of delivering the AA message, the meetings have a latent function which is at least as important in terms of helping the alcoholic to achieve and maintain sobriety. Gellman, along with several other students of this group, refers to AA as organization therapy.[17-21] He posits that "the structure and processes of the total social system of the organization" are central to the therapy offered to the alcoholic. The goal of the fellowship is to provide an atmosphere that is so congenial that the alcoholic will replace his old peer group of drinking friends with this new abstinent one. Since the individual is told that the disease of alcoholism is a permanent affliction and that he can never drink another drop of alcohol, he is encouraged to make permanent friendships within the group. In this way, AA is a fellowship in the literal sense. As Maxwell states,

> *In countless ways, AA provides the rewards of satisfying social activities to replace the rewards previously sought in a drinking group, or simply sought in the bottle itself.*[22]

Sponsorship. It is generally believed that one of the best ways of assuring successful affiliation with AA is through sponsorship. There are two major ways by which a prospective member can acquire a sponsor: a response to a Twelfth Step call or an appearance at a meeting. It is the sponsors' responsibility to introduce their charges to the AA program, to encourage them to go to meetings, to be available as often as possible for support, and in general to aid the successful resocialization of the alcoholic. Once the new members become stable for several months, it is expected that this relationship will be attenuated and that they themselves will become a sponsor.

Affiliation. As stated in Tradition 3, the only membership requirement is the desire to stop drinking. Therefore, it is expected that AA would be representative of sub-groups within the population of alcoholics, such as race and sex. However, it has been argued that AA is a voluntary association of sorts with an ideology that is not consistent with the values of either the white lower class or black subcultures. In effect, it is suggested that AA is largely a white middle class organization, like so many other well-entrenched groups in our society.

Several studies of the affiliation process lend support to the hypothesis that alcoholics with at least middle class occupational backgrounds are disproportionately represented.[23-28] The explanation for this is that AA is imbued with the Protestant ethic, emphasizing such goals as emotional control, pragmatism, inner strength, and godliness.[29] As Trice states, "Although AA is composed of deviants as far as drinking is concerned, it is characteristic of the general American scene from which it emerged."[30] Thus it is argued from a clearly subcultural perspective that the goals espoused by AA are inimical to the value orientations of the white lower class and black lifestyles.

However, there are also several studies which do not support this hypothesis, indicating that socioeconomic status is of little importance in determining affiliation or degree of activity.[31-33] In fact, it is suggested by such studies that AA is a successful bridge across class barriers. There are a number of black AA groups in the larger cities of Pennsylvania, and some of these, such as one in a lower class area of Erie, are comprised of lower class blacks with an admixture of other racial groups. In an interview, the leader of this group expressed the feeling that the heavy concentration of white middle class people in AA was an historical accident, resulting from the origin of AA in the white middle class (Bill W. was a New York stockbroker and Dr. Bob an Akron surgeon). They tended to attract others like themselves. But he felt that the AA approach and philosophy were entirely congenial to lower class blacks and whites, as demonstrated by the experience of his group. What was required was an AA leader working in a lower class area.

At one point, the research team contemplated making a special study of this issue. The reasoning was that if AA were not congenial to all sociocultural groups, its equivalent might have to be developed. The study's projected first step was to have been a democratic survey of the AA membership in one area of Pennsylvania to determine its composition. However, it rapidly became clear that AA would not permit such a study, and that its anonymity precluded the study being carried out. This invulnerability to careful study is both a strength and a weakness for AA, and is one which is shared with its offspring in the drug treatment area, Synanon.

AA and Pennsylvania Treatment Facilities

Out of 80 facilities, 53, or 66%, had at least one AA group associated with them. By association, it is meant that an AA group has an ongoing relationship with the program and conducts regularly scheduled meetings on the premises. Out of a total of 6,805 patients in treatment, 3,344 (49%) were involved with an AA chapter as members. (This figure is probably an under-representation, since two program directors stated that they did not know how many of their patients were involved in AA.) No large differences were found according to population size. Urban programs were defined as those located in either Philadelphia or Allegheny Counties, while other programs were located in suburban, small city, or rural areas. Regardless of the population size of the area of location,[16] about two-thirds of all programs were affiliated with AA. However, there was some difference with respect to numbers of alcoholics affiliated with AA. In programs located in small cities and rural areas, approximately half of the patients, 50.6% and 54.1%, respectively, were associated with at least one AA group. In contrast, urban programs had the lowest proportion (41.8%), while suburban programs had the highest proportion of patients affiliated with AA (67.1%).

It is evident that AA represents a major method of treating alcoholism in Pennsylvania. Our survey indicates its influence is pervasive. Not only does it have a vast membership in its own activities outside of formal treatment programs, but it interacts on an ongoing basis with the majority of programs. In addition, 27% of the total treatment staff of Commonwealth programs are recovered alcoholics, many of whom are products of AA. Alcoholics Anonymous' philosophy dominates many programs completely, and pervades the entire treatment system.

Alcoholics Anonymous has a number of significant advantages. It provides for continuity of care after the individual has been released from a residential program. Through two related but independent organizations, Al-Anon and Alateen, the spouses, children, and friends of alcoholics share problems, advice, and support in dealing with them. In addition, alcoholics are given a viable alternative to the loneliness and isolation that generally accompanies alcoholism; they are provided with a diverse set of sober alcoholics and activities from which to build a satisfying and lasting social life. Lastly, it is a completely voluntary organization, with absolutely no cost to the taxpayer.

Thus, AA can and should continue to play a major role in the Commonwealth's approach to alcoholism. Yet its very size and success pose a number of important problems. It may be accepted as factual that the alcoholic population is diverse and contains many different subgroups. While the AA method may be satisfactory for many alcoholics, it is not likely to be suitable for everyone. This would present no problem if many AA adherents were tolerant of alternative approaches. Such is not the case. Like so many organizations with a strong ideological base, professional organizations not excluded, AA members are often totally intolerant of alternative treatment approaches. They often argue that in the face of their success other approaches are unnecessary, forgetting that their organization has proven largely impervious to empirical study and that, in terms of current research capabilities, the efficacy of AA has never been carefully studied, much less definitely demonstrated.[34] As one student of the organization has remarked, "... AA merits more understanding than the current state of knowledge about it affords."[35] It may be expected that if the Commonwealth supports diverse treatment approaches to alcoholism, including the use of chemotherapy and of behavioral modification methods to promote controlled drinking for some populations, AA members will object strenuously.

For all that, Commonwealth and its citizens owe an incalculable debt to the courage and determination of this remarkable and dedicated group. These people have been the true frontiersmen in this dark wilderness of the human spirit. But for their persistence, there might not now exist any serious approach to the problem of alcoholism.

References

1. Profile of an AA meeting. Alcoholics Anonymous World Services, Inc. New York, 1972.
2. Leach, B. Does Alcoholics Anonymous really work? *In:* Bourne, P.G. and Fox, R. (eds.). *Alcoholism: Progress in research and treatment.* New York: Academic Press, 1973, pp. 245-284.
3. *Alcoholics Anonymous comes of age.* New York: Alcoholics Anonymous World Service, Inc. 1957.
4. Eister, A.W. *Drawing-room conversion.* Durham, N.C.: Duke University Press, 1950.
5. Clark, W.H. *The Oxford group: Its history and significance.* New York: Bookman Associates, 1951.
6. Eister, *op.cit.*
7. Eister, *Ibid.*
8. *Alcoholics Anonymous comes of age. op. cit.* pp. 62-63.
9. Chafetz, M.D. and Demone, H.W., Jr. *Alcoholism and society.* New York: Oxford University Press, 1962.
10. *Alcoholics Anonymous comes of age. op,cit.*
11. Gellman, I.P. *The sober alcoholic.* New Haven: College and University Press, 1964.
12. Trice, H.M. and Roman, P.M. Delabeling, relabeling, and Alcoholics Anonymous. *Social Problems, 17* (4): 538-546, Spring 1970.
13. Chafetz and Demone, *op.cit.*
14. Ritchie, O.W. A sociohistorical survey of Alcoholics Anonymous. *Journal of Studies on Alcohol, 9:* 119-156, 1948.
15. Gellman, *op.cit.*
16. Gellman, *Ibid.*
17. Gellman, *Ibid.*

18. Maxwell, M.A. Alcoholics Anonymous: An interpretation. *In:* Pittman, D.J. *Alcoholism,* New York: Harper & Row, 1971, pp. 211-222.

19. Trice, H.M. Alcoholics Anonymous. *Annals of the American Academy of Political and Social Sciences,* January 1958, pp. 108-116.

20. Chafetz and Demone, *op.cit.*

21. Kessel, N. and Walton, H. *Alcoholism,* Middlesex, England: Penguin Books, Ltd., 1965.

22. Maxwell, *op.cit.* p. 220.

23. Trice, H.M. A study of the process of affiliation with Alcoholics Anonymous. *Journal of Studies on Alcohol, 18:* 39-54, 1957.

24. Trice, H.M. The affiliation motive and readiness to join Alcoholics Anonymous. *Journal of Studies on Alcohol, 20:* 313-320, 1959.

25. Chafetz and Demone, *op.cit.*

26. Trice, Alcoholics Anonymous. *op.cit.*

27. Lemert, E.W. *Alcohol and the Northwest Coast Indians.* Berkeley, California: University of California Press, 1954.

28. Schmidt, W., Smart, R.G., and Moss, M.K. *Social class and the treatment of alcoholism.* Toronto: University of Toronto Press, 1968.

29. Chafetz and Demone, *op.cit.*

30. Trice, Alcoholics Anonymous. *op.cit.* p. 115.

31. Lofland, J.F. and Lejeune, R.A. Initial interaction of newcomers in AA: A field experiment in class symbols and socialization. *Social Problems, 8:* 103-111, Fall 1960.

32. Murphy, M.M. Values stressed by two social class levels at meetings of Alcoholics Anonymous. *Journal of Studies on Alcohol, 14:* 576-85, 1953.

33. Trice, H.M. and Roman, P.M. Sociopsychological predictors of affiliation with Alcoholics Anonymous. *Social Psychiatry, 5:* (1) 51-59, 1970.

34. For a comprehensive summary of the findings and analysis of the limitations of four studies of abstinence and relapses among AA members, see Leach, *op.cit.*

35. Leach, *Ibid.*

Chapter 14

Rescue Missions

No survey of the treatment of alcoholism would be complete without mention of one of the oldest and best known forms of alcoholism care in the United States—the religious organizations generally referred to as missions. While missions vary in terms of organizational affiliation, their general approach to alcoholism and its treatment is quite similar. The site-visiting team did not attempt to visit all Pennsylvania missions. However we did visit representatives of each of perhaps the best known missions; those affiliated with the International Union of Gospel Missions and the Harbor Light centres of the Salvation Army. Even though these represent a fraction of the total number of such facilities,* we felt that the others would be sufficiently similar as to make this sample adequate for the purpose of description.**

Salvation Army Missions

The Salvation Army has a long history of offering aid to anyone in need of either spiritual or material uplifting. Basically, its approach consists of a practical application of Christian ideals in order to offer help to the

* For example, Blumberg, Shipley, and Shandler report 17 missions and quasi-missions in Philadelphia in the mid-1960s.[16]

** The four missions discussed in this chapter are not included in the 80 programs treated elsewhere in this report. The reason for this is that the missions differ so radically from the other forms of treatment that it would be inappropriate to categorize them together.

victims of a variety of social problems. It is one of the many social reform movements deriving inspiration from evangelical Protestantism. Such social reform groups were prevalent in Britain and the United States in the late 19th century. Unlike most of these groups, the Salvation Army has successfully weathered changes in the social climate. From its inception in 1865, the Salvation Army has directed its efforts toward helping the alcoholic, along with the poor, the elderly, the homeless, and the handicapped.

In 1890 General William Booth, the founder of the Salvation Army, wrote the original Salvationist treatise on alcoholism and its treatment, *In Darkest England and the Way Out.* It was based on his experiences in dealing with the drunkards of late 19th century London. Contrary to popular opinion, Booth's conception of alcoholism was surprisingly similar to the 20th century disease model of Jellinek, Alcoholics Anonymous, and others. Booth states, "It is a disease often inherited, always developed by indulgence, but as clearly a disease as opthalmia or stone."[2] In addition, Booth recognized the loss of control which is regarded by some as one of the distinguishing characteristics of alcoholism. "The drunkard (struggling alone) promises and vows in vain. Insatiable craving controls him. He cannot get away. Unless delivered by an Almighty hand, he will drink himself into the grave."[3] He also included a social component among the etiological factors; he felt that the dehumanizing effects of living in a slum environment were instrumental in exacerbating the addiction process.

Booth's relatively modern definition of alcoholism has apparently been tempered to some extent by the more traditional views of some of his followers. To many Salvationists, alcoholism represents a moral failing for which the individual is entirely responsible. Since God created man in his own image, it is sinful to defile the body or the spirit in any way, including the ingestion of alcohol. Therefore, alcohol consumption of any kind is considered a sin. While not everyone who drinks will become an alcoholic, the risk is too great to take the chance. The individual is an alcoholic by choice; had he not taken that first drink, he would not now be in this sorry state.[4] Thus, the Salvation Army has had a range of conceptualizations of alcoholism, from an early version of the disease concept to the moral model.

This eclecticism was demonstrated by the directors of the two Harbor Light centres visited in the present survey. In one case, alcoholism was defined as a combination of a moral failing and a progressive process of addiction; in the other, the conception was in terms of both a moral component and a symptom of an underlying personality disorder. While in both instances the element of individual moral responsibility was present, the more recent secular views of alcoholism were also represented.

Judging from the range of definitions of the problem that has been espoused by the Salvation Army, one could expect an equally eclectic approach with respect to treatment goals. The obvious corollary to the disease conception of the etiology of alcoholism is abstinence as a treatment goal. This is, in disease theory, a prerequisite for any other therapeutic objective. However, not only is it a goal for the treatment of the alcoholic, according to the Salvation Army, but it represents the only sensible form of prevention. If one does not drink, one cannot become an alcoholic. Therefore, the Salvation Army has historically been a strong advocate of abstinence as a general societal goal. Both Salvation Army respondents stated that abstinence was a major treatment objective.

While alcoholics must always aim for abstinence as a long-range goal, they will be unable to accomplish this unless they achieve the overriding objective of treatment: salvation. Since man is by his very nature weak, he must surrender his will to a higher power in order to draw strength and sustenance. Only in this way can the individual even begin to travel the long, arduous road of maintaining abstinence and rejoining society. While this goal closely resembles that of Alcoholics Anonymous, it differs in that the Salvation Army defines the higher power specifically as Jesus Christ. By allowing Christ to come into one's life through one's faith in Him, one will receive the divine guidance that is absolutely essential to the accomplishment of any goal in life, including abstinence. While certainly any course of treatment should avail itself of the advances of modern science, according to the Salvation Army permanent rehabilitation can only take place through faith.

This program of salvation by divine grace through faith is taken directly from Protestant theology. It is an application of the philosophy of salvation through faith rather than work. Alcoholics may devote themselves tirelessly to a strict therapeutic regime, but unless they accept Christ, their work will be for naught. In addition the emphasis on a direct relationship between man and God, as illustrated in the prescription to "let Christ into your life," is another direct outgrowth of the individualism that is a central theme in Protestantism.[5] One of our Salvation Army respondents clearly stated that communication with God was a specific goal; "Jesus Christ is the answer." The other responded in terms of a change in lifestyle, a new direction in life.

The actual programs organized by the Salvation Army have been quite varied. One of the most colorful efforts was a series of events known as Boozers' Days. Just prior to World War I, the Army decided that it needed a dramatic means of extending its spiritual message to alcoholics. Hence, for several years on Thanksgiving Day and Washington's Birthday, round-up crews were dispatched to the various tenderloin areas of New York at four in the morning. The drunks were brought by bus to Army headquarters, where they were bombarded by testimonies from recovered alcoholics. The hope was that by hearing the success stories of their former fellow alcoholics, they would be sufficiently impressed to undergo a spiritual conversion. This event was repeated three times on each Boozers' Day.[6] However the practice was phased out after several years.

A more recent program of treatment is a set of steps known as "Road Markers."[7] Developed in the early 1940s by Envoy J. Stanley Sheppard, the influence of AA, which at that time was beginning to rise to prominence, is pervasive. The main difference is that the higher power is defined specifically as Christ rather than being left to individual interpretation.

Road Markers on "The Way Back"

The alcoholic must realize that he is unable to control his addiction and that his life is completely disorganized.

He must acknowledge that only God, his Creator, can recreate him as a decent man.

He must let God through Jesus Christ rule his life and resolve to live according to His will.

He must realize that alcohol addiction is only a symptom of basic defects in his thinking and living, and that the proper use of every talent he possesses is impaired by his enslavement.

He should make public confession, to God and man, of past wrongdoings and be willing to ask God for guidance in the future.

He should make restitution to all whom he has willfully and knowingly wronged.

He should realize that he is human and subject to error and that no advance is made by covering up a mistake; he should admit failure and profit by experience.

Since, through prayer and forgiveness he has found Christ, he must continue prayerful contact with Him and seek constantly to know His will.

Because the Salvation Army believes that the personal touch and example are the most vital forces in applying the principles of Christianity, he should be made to work continuously not only for his own salvation but to help effect the salvation of others like himself.

The Salvation Army holds an eternal faith in the all-conquering power of God—a conviction that no matter how bad a man is or how far he has fallen, there still is good in him. Our task is to find that spark and fan it into a flame. This will call for intelligent understanding of human nature, sympathy, tact, firmness, tenderness, common sense—and an appreciation of the limitations of the alcoholic; unceasing vigilance, continuity of effort and the consistency of personal example by the Salvationist.

The extent of the application of these rules in the programs visited by the survey team is highly questionable. Neither of our respondents made any reference to them.

The actual program as it appears to operate on a daily basis has three major components. The first, and most important, is what the Army refers to as "therapy of faith." This consists of a regime of morning devotions, evening prayer meetings, and individual prayer sessions. Anyone is invited to attend the prayer meetings. As in any religious service, all activity is directed toward the creation of an intense emotional atmosphere that is collectively experienced. While the manifest function is to convey the message of salvation, the latent function is to draw individuals out of their own private existence and into the group.[8] However, unlike many other forms of religious gathering, there is almost no ritual. This illustrates the strong connection between the Army and Protestantism with respect to the latter's reaction against the ritualism of the Catholic Church. Through hymns, testimonies, and constant encouragement to find Christ, it is hoped that a number of the members of the audience will undergo the joyful experience of conversion. Without the discovery of Christ, all else is impossible.

The second component is the food and shelter that are provided after the prayer meeting. The third component is work. At Harbor Light centres, the staff attempts to find the men "spot" jobs in the community, as soon as they are able to work.* They are expected to pay a small fee for room, board, and other services, and to rejoin the community as quickly as possible.** However, at the centres visited, the men tended to live there for fairly long periods, an average of three months at one and six months at the other. Again, this emphasis on work illustrates the close connection between the Army and Protestantism. A major theme in the latter is the moral incumbency upon every individual to diligently pursue an honest occupation for the purpose of carrying out God's will. Known as a "calling," it is one of the few ways in which an individual may know that he has been selected for salvation.[9]

Perhaps what the Salvation Army is best known for is its history as a permanent fixture of the skid rows of most American and some European cities. Along with flophouses, bars, cheap restaurants, all-night movies, and warehouses, the Salvation Army's Harbor Light and Men's Social Service centres have been a fixture of tenderloin sections

* One out of six men in one program and three out of 10 in the other were employed full-time; both programs referred their clients to the State Bureau of Vocational Rehabilitation.

** At the Men's Social Service centres, which also treat alcoholics along with the handicapped, there is a greater tendency to live and work at the centre on a more permanent basis than in the Harbor Light centres.

TABLE 1

Characteristics of Residents at Salvation Army Harbor Light Centres and Rescue Missions

	No. (All male)	Whites	Non-whites	Age of youngest	Age of oldest	Average age	Educational level	Occupational level	No. Employed
Harbor Light A	10	10	0	49	72	55	9th gr. or less	Derelict	3
Harbor Light B	6	5	1	24	62	45	H.S. graduate	Skilled blue collar	1
Rescue Mission A	14	11	3	40	70	55	9th gr. or less	Unskilled blue collar	0
Rescue Mission B	100	93	7	24	74	50	H.S. attendance	Unskilled blue collar	0

	From same county as program	Alcohol abused	Major secondary drug
Harbor Light A	10	Wine	Amphetamines
Harbor Light B	6	Wine	Tranquillizers
Rescue Mission A	3	Wine	Tranquillizers
Rescue Mission B	10	Combination	Don't know

TABLE 2

Characteristics of Staff at Salvation Army
Harbor Light Centres and Rescue Missions

	Full-time staff	White	Non-white	Director's education	College grads or above	Recovered alcoholics	Part-time staff	Part-time physicians
Harbor Light A	4	4	0	H.S. attendance	0	2	0	2
Harbor Light B	5	5	0	Minister	0	1	1	0
Rescue Mission A	11	11	0	Minister	1	0	0	0
Rescue Mission B	10	9	1	Minister	0	0	4	0

for a century. In skid row parlance, the Army's operations are (perhaps affectionately) referred to as "Sally." The facilities visited in the present survey were relatively new; one admitted the first patient to its present facility in 1956 and the other in 1957. (One was located in a former office building and the other in a former hardware store.)

The patient population is homogenous: homeless men having little education, few job skills, and long histories of excessive drinking and general instability.[10] Typically, they have been through the "revolving door" of the criminal justice system, in which they are picked up by the police as public inebriates, spend a night or two in the drunk tank, appear before a judge briefly, and are quickly released back to the street. The recognition of the futility of this cycle has resulted in the abandonment of the practice in some areas.

While the alcoholics seen by one of the Harbor Light centres conformed to this typification, those seen in the other did not. The latter appeared to be younger, better educated, and more skilled (see Table 1). In general, though, the men were of relatively low educational and occupational achievement.

It is reported that some centres employ mental health professionals, such as social workers, psychiatrists, and vocational counselors.[11,12] But this was not the case in the facilities visited. None of the staff, including the director, of either program had college degrees, even though one program employed two part-time physicians (see Table 2). Given the manifestly religious orientation of the Harbor Light program, it is not unexpected that the staff had little in the way of mental health training. Anyone who has a strong faith in God and the desire to help others has all the necessary qualifications, according to the precepts of the Army.

In terms of recommendations as to what the Commonwealth should do to alleviate the problem of alcoholism, both directors emphasized the importance of education. They stated that the responsibility of educating children on the problem of alcoholism should be taken by the public schools, and the education process must begin at the primary level. The other recommendation, which was made by one program, was that it was immoral for the state to be engaged in the business of selling liquor, particularly for the purpose of increased revenue. This reflects the moral stance that the Army has taken toward the etiology of alcoholism, in which the consumption of alcohol is viewed as one of its root causes.

In conclusion, the Salvation Army has played a significant role in the care of skid row alcoholics for the past century. Throughout its history, it has remained a haven for problem drinkers who have few resources upon which to draw and who have found other treatment programs either unavailable or unwilling to care for them. The Army's approach is strongly moralistic, but the enlightened views of the founder,

General Booth, have encouraged some appreciation of recent advances in the treatment of alcoholism.

Rescue Missions

The rescue missions that were visited for this survey were both affiliates of the International Union of Gospel Missions. The official year of the Union's inception is 1872, when the first rescue mission was founded in New York by Jerry McAuley, a recovered alcoholic who was a convert to evangelical Protestantism. It was incorporated in 1913 into a confederation of semi-autonomous missions. Currently, there are 350 missions throughout the world. The role of the I.U.G.M. is to provide training for mission workers, conduct public relations, and develop standards for care. In keeping with its philosophy of "seeking the last, the least, and the lost," this organization provides a diversity of services, including sheltered workshops, children's homes, alcoholic clinics, and family counseling. Similar to the Salvation Army, the alcoholic is viewed by the missions as another unfortunate, along with the poor, the elderly, and the handicapped, who is deserving of the strength and guidance of the Christian way of life.

In contrast to the Salvation Army, the rescue missions define alcoholism solely in moral terms. It is a natural consequence of indulging in alcohol, which is a sin of the most serious order. The rescue missions reject outright all notions of alcoholism as a disease, and they present the following elaborate argument to prove their point.[13]

Is Alcoholism a Disease?

The problem: not alcoholism, but alcohol. There could be no problem of alcoholism without alcohol.
If it is a disease, it is a disease without germ or virus.
If it is a disease, it is the only disease that is self-inflicted.
If it is a disease, it is the only disease contracted by an act of the will. This is not true of any other sickness.
If it is a disease, it is the only disease that is bottled and sold over the counter for a profit.
If it is a disease, it is the only disease that brings in tax revenue for the government, state, county, and city.
If it is a disease, it is the only disease that takes thousands of outlets in every town and city to spread it.
If it is a disease, it is the only disease that they spend four to five hundred million dollars a year to spread it.
If it is a disease, it is the only disease that provokes crime, and corrupts our courts and law enforcement officials.
If it is a disease, it is the only disease that turns our boys into criminals and our girls into prostitutes.

> *If it is a disease, it is the only disease that will cause a father to go home and take his baby by the heels and beat its brains out.*
> *If it is a disease, it is the only disease that will cause a mother to desert her children, and leave them on the mercy of the world.*
> *If it is a disease, it is the only disease that will take the clothes from their back, shoes from their feet, and bread from their mouths.*
> *If it is a disease, it is the only disease that is bottled and sold, causing our reform schools, jails, and mental institutions to be filled.*
> *If it is a disease, it is the only disease that is given for a Christmas present.*

The rescue missions posit that the disease concept is an intellectual rationalization for behavior that is determined by the choice of the individual. As such it is an abdication of responsibility and a denial of its real cause, the sin of alcohol consumption. Thus, alcoholism is both self-inflicted and dependent on the use of alcohol, which is pervasive in our society. As expected, the directors of both rescue missions visited defined alcoholism solely in terms of sin.

From this conception of alcoholism, it follows that the goal of treatment should be twofold: abstinence and the surrender of the will to God. As in the Salvation Army, not only is abstinence an obvious goal for the alcoholic, but it is also a value that society in general should seek to attain. However, this is impossible unless every individual in the community accepts Christ into his life. Again, as in the Salvation Army, the philosophy of salvation through faith alone that is a major component of Protestant theology is the ideological foundation upon which the rescue mission program is based. Both mission directors interviewed indicated that their principal treatment objective was to help the men establish a close relationship with God that would change their lives. In fact, one mission director erected a 22-foot high electric sign at the main entrance to the town in which his mission was located, reading "CHRIST IS THE ANSWER"!

While the rescue mission movement has not produced a set of rules for recovery like the "Road Markers" of the Salvation Army, their actual program is quite similar to that of the Army. There is a threefold format—prayer, food and shelter, and work. The first two components are virtually identical to the Salvation Army. However, in the rescue mission the work is done largely inside the mission rather than in the form of "spot" jobs in the community. In fact, the missions are actually a type of sheltered workshop. In one mission visited, the men were involved in the repair of items donated to the thrift shop. In the other, there was a large newspaper baling operation, complete with baling machines, a warehouse, and a fleet of trucks. At the time of the interview, none of the men in either mission was employed outside, nor referred to the Bureau of Vocational Rehabilitation. Thus, work did not appear to be viewed in a community context, but rather as an integral part of the activities conducted on the grounds of the mission.

Rescue missions, much like the Salvation Army, have been a permanent fixture of skid row areas for many years. The missions visited, both of which were located in small cities, admitted their first patients at the turn of the century. They were located in buildings that had been constructed especially for use as rescue missions. However, over the years, both had expanded into a complex of buildings in order to accommodate their work operations and thrift shops.

The men living at the rescue mission seemed to conform to the usual characteristics attributed to inhabitants of skid row, in terms of age, education, and occupational skills (see Table 1). In addition, the men at the rescue missions seemed considerably more geographically mobile than was the case at the Salvation Army. Only a handful came from the county in which the mission was located, and a substantial portion came from outside Pennsylvania. This, in conjunction with the fact that the average length of stay at each mission was only four weeks, conjures up the stereotypical image of skid row bums who tour the country at the hospitality of the rescue missions.

Judging from the rescue missions' approach to alcoholism, one would not expect them to be staffed by mental health professionals. Since alcoholism is a moral failing, there is little need for people whose competence lies outside the spiritual realm. Each of the missions visited had close to a dozen full-time staff, none of whom were college graduates; the directors were both ordained ministers in one of the evangelical sects; neither program employed a physician on even a part-time basis (see Table 2).

In contrast to other programs, including the Salvation Army, recommendations from the rescue missions were not in the form of proposed activities for state government. Rather they proclaimed that the only recommendation for the treatment of alcoholism is salvation. This is logical since problems that affect human beings are not caused by social factors which are external to individuals or psychological processes within the individual, but rather they are the result of the failure to accept Christ. Without this, according to the missions, governmental efforts are for naught.

Conclusion

The ideological basis, approach, and program of the Salvation Army and of the rescue missions affiliated with the International Union of Gospel Missions have generally been grouped together as one aspect of the societal response to alcoholism. Siegler *et al* labeled this the "dry moral model" (dry refers to the abstinence prescription).[14] Their single-minded devotion to salvation, prayer, and abstinence with little attention to the social and psychological factors that are thought by mental health professionals to be the causes of alcoholism has prompted a good deal of questioning by these same professionals as to the efficacy of the moral model. It is asserted that their interpretations of the conditions predisposing an individual to excessive drinking are so simplistic as to render their approach ineffective.[15]

However, it must be remembered that these centres, at the very least, provide for the physical necessities of food, clothing, and shelter. At the most, they may even effect permanent rehabilitation for some alcoholics. Historically, they have provided services to a population of alcoholics that was often unreached by more conventional types of treatment. If the Salvation Army and rescue missions have accomplished nothing else, this fact alone would justify their existence. That they may well have accomplished more is suggested by a survey of skid row men in which over half felt that the missions helped the men and a sixth gave a mixed yes-no response.[16]

Given the current state of alcoholism treatment, any group which is perceived as being helpful by 70% of its target population would be difficult to dismiss out of hand. It is also far too easy to forget that this significant service is being rendered without causing any draw upon tax revenues. Moreover, the quasi-domiciliary level of care offered by the missions may be quite appropriate in terms of the reasonable therapeutic expectations one may entertain for many of their clients. To be sure, the full potential of many residents may never be reached owing to the routinized processing of the mission, but much the same criticism could be made of most treatment programs. And certainly the survey of treatment programs suggests that the supportive services being provided by the missions in terms of food and shelter are not readily available throughout the state.

Thus, no sober thought of phasing out the missions should be entertained at least until equally supportive alternatives are available. Moreover, our limited survey suggests that missions cannot properly be lumped together, but that there are at least two major varieties entertaining rather different assumptions and goals on the nature of the problem and its solution. This suggests that further study of and familiarity with such operations might eventually lead to a closer integration of their services with those of others striving toward the same goals.

References

1. Clinebell, H.J. How religion has been used to help homeless alcoholics. *Understanding and Counseling the Alcoholic.* New York: Abingdon Press, 1956, pp. 69-93.

2. Booth, W. *In darkest England and the way out.* Atlanta, Ga.: The Salvation Army, 1942, p. 48.

3. *The Salvation Army and the alcoholic.* New York: National Research Bureau of the Salvation Army, 1948, p. 8.

4. *Ibid.*

5. Weber, M. *The Protestant ethic and the spirit of capitalism.* Talcott Parsons (trans.), New York: Charles Scribner's Sons, 1958.

6. The Salvation Army and the alcoholic, *op.cit.*

7. *Ibid.*

8. Durkheim, E. *The elementary forms of the religious life.* J.W. Swain (trans.), New York: Free Press, 1965.

9. Weber, *op.cit.*

10. Lovald, K. and Stub, H.R. The revolving door: Reactions of chronic drunkenness offenders to court sanctions. *Journal of Criminal Law, Criminology and Police Science, 59* (4): 525-30, 1968.

11. Clinebell, *op.cit.*

12. Katz, L. The Salvation Army men's social service centers; I. Program. *Journal of Studies on Alcohol, 25:* 324-332, 1964.

13. So you are convinced that alcoholism is a disease! United Mission Services, Inc., P.O. Box 36606, Houston, Texas. No. T-5.

14. Siegler, M., Osmond, H., and Newell, S. Models of alcoholism. *Journal of Studies on Alcohol,* 29: 571-591, 1968.

15. Clinebell, *op.cit.*

16. Blumberg, L., Shipley, T.E., and Shandler, I. *Skid row and its alternatives: Research and recommendations from Philadelphia.* Philadelphia: Temple University Press, 1973, p. 89.

Chapter 15

Education Programs

One of the major problems in the treatment of alcoholism has been and continues to be the absence of an adequate and generally-recognized conceptual model for education and prevention programs. As discussed in an earlier chapter, excessive drinking has been defined variously in terms of moral/ethical, medical, legal, psychiatric, social welfare, or public health perspectives, but rarely has it been viewed as involving all of these systems concurrently. Current social responses tend to reflect a relative over-emphasis upon the medical model to the neglect of other perspectives.

The search for an understanding of the causes of alcohol-related problems and for modes of intervention has included considerations of heredity; of the structural, biochemical, and physiological attributes of the human body; of the characteristics of personality; or of the influences of society, culture, and environment. Rarely has this search assumed an interaction of all these variables. Most programs for coping with alcohol problems have emphasized the unique and directly-related aspects, and have given too little attention to development primary prevention models for implementation in the schools and community.

What are the major types of programs in the field of alcohol education? To what extent have they been successful in reducing the incidence of problem drinking? Since these questions are of direct relevance to a comprehensive alcoholism program, a member of the survey team visited several school districts in the suburban Philadelphia area. The team also sought the advice of many administrators and educators within the Commonwealth and consulted the program directors of school and community drug and alcohol prevention programs. We found that virtually all efforts in drug education can be placed into one of the four following categories: (1) general education programs for the purpose of disseminating information, often involving hospital personnel and the police as well as teachers trained as "instant" experts; (2) community-based information programs; (3) group process training programs for teachers and administrators, designed to improve channels for communication in the schools; and (4) sensitivity or group dynamics training programs for students, involving values clarification, peer group counseling, rap or drop-in centres, and other such methods, aimed at effective rather than cognitive education.

General Information Programs

Initial attempts at the development of education programs have primarily focused on supplying information to the general population about the negative effects of alcohol abuse. Such programs assume that all segments of the society must first receive extensive amounts of drug information in order to permit individuals to make informed decisions about drug abuse. Recipients are taught about the medical aspects of alcoholism and exposed to assembly programs and small group discussions that deal with the legal, political, ethical, moral, and religious implications of alcohol abuse. These programs often feature testimony by recovered alcoholics and employ "scare" tactics in an attempt to curtail usage. Participants in these programs are informed of the demographic characteristics of alcoholics, the types of alcohol frequently abused, the frequency of use, the settings in which alcohol was used, common personality characteristics of the user, and the deviant manner in which users frequently behave.

Discussions of the social and psychological complications of alcohol abuse often address such issues as whether society should accept alcoholism as a permanent condition and the consequences of this acceptance. The programs also focus on the legal aspects of abuse by considering such questions as: Do laws have to be changed to suit the changing characteristics of society? At what stage and to what degree should the legal system become involved in dealing with major social problems? Needless to say, these discussions often reflect the values of the educators planning the programs.

Specifically, general information programs are concerned with improving and providing support for school programs. In order to accomplish this goal, programs sponsored by hospitals, police forces, and civic organizations have initiated training and counseling programs for administrators, teachers, school nurses, school psychologists, and guidance counselors. Agency consultants, often trained as "instant" experts through their attendance at a single course or workshop at a hospital or university, may assist school districts in the development of in-service courses, workshops, and teachers' one-day conferences on drug abuse. Other activities include sending information bulletins to school districts and preparing pamphlets for teachers, telling them how to diagnose alcoholism and drug abuse among their students. Underlying all these programs is the assumption that clear and unbiased information constitutes the essential means for effective alcohol prevention. Their basic premise is that when hard facts are made available, attitudes toward drugs and alcohol will change; attitude change will then result in a reduction of drug experimentation among students.

Community-Based Health Education Programs

Community information programs, the second major type of program, are based on the assumption that alcohol abuse is primarily a manifestation of poor health practices in general and "improper" attitudes and habits about health matters in our society in particular. According to this orientation, prevention will only be accomplished when students recognize the positive effects that accrue from good health practices to themselves, their families, the community, and the society at large. Such programs expect the schools to cooperate with community organizations in an effort to improve the physical health of students through health education programs that present scientific information and research findings about alcoholism and related topics. The best of these programs are designed to permit students to raise questions, formulate answers, and arrive at sound conclusions concerning such issues as human sexuality, venereal disease, alcoholism, drug abuse, and smoking. Similar to general information programs, it is the basic assumption of health education programs that if students obtain factual information they will develop a sense of personal and social responsibility such that they will elect not to use drugs or alcohol, engage in premarital sex, or smoke. But in this instance the emphasis is upon the positive (health) and the perspective is broad, rather than being both negative (ill health) and specific.

Preventive efforts include the use of speakers at such gatherings as school assemblies, student meetings, adult education programs, church conferences, and in-service workshops for administrators, teachers, counselors, doctors, nurses, clergy, and the police. The speakers frequently report conditions of drug and alcohol abuse as they have encountered them, and propose projects or present assembly programs on the topic. A number of community-based programs have relied heavily on the expertise of general practitioners, psychologists, members of Alcoholics Anonymous, and individuals with special training in youth work.

Group Process Training for Administrators and Teachers

The third type of program focuses on group process training for school administrators, guidance personnel, and teachers. Efforts of this kind represent attempts to improve the ability to relate to others by increasing the individual's understanding of both the strains he experiences in his role and those to which the students are subject. Such programs also attempt to deal with feelings and motivations. One goal of these programs is to create greater "openness"in administrator-teacher-student interactions. Another is to allow teachers to feel more comfortable in assigning more responsibility for learning and personal growth to students in the hope that their stake in their own development and that of the existing system in general will be increased. The assumption on which group process training is based is that deviant behavior such as alcohol abuse will be reduced if educators become sensitized to the ways in which their general attitudes and behaviors, as well as those concerning drug and alcohol abuse, affect their students. Improved understanding and communication will reduce stress, and hence the need for deviant behavior.

Teachers and administrators typically meet in small groups to discuss readings in such areas as group dynamics and the peer-group subculture as they both relate to alcohol abuse and to other forms of deviant behavior. Discussions follow in which the group generally experiences an initial phase involving dependency on a group leader and an atmosphere of confusion and uneasiness. In the second phase, attention is directed to the examination of adult behavior in schools and its effect on students. Finally, participants experiment with new forms of behavior and are exposed to immediate feedback concerning the ways in which their behavior is perceived by others.

It should be emphasized that group dynamics programs represent one of the earliest attempts to deal affectively, rather than cognitively, with the alcoholism problem. However, while changes in staff attitudes may arise from increased self-understanding, self-esteem, and increased communication skills, the available evidence unfortunately provides no support for the idea that improving the environment of the school without also taking into account other social influences on students will stem the ride of alcohol abuse.

Sensitivity Training

Programs in the fourth category are designed to address primary causes of alcohol abuse behavior and attempt to uncover underlying "casual" factors. We noted earlier that many studies have tried to identify environmental factors associated with alcohol abuse, such as lack of family cohesiveness, peer group pressures, identity crises in adolescence, the rejection of authority, alienation, and the elusive "communications gap" between adults and children. A logical extension of this thinking is that countervailing environmental influences favoring positive behaviors can be brought to bear upon populations at risk through the medium of the school. These programs typically assume that appropriate educational experiences will help students to discover and control their own motivations and to seek more socially-acceptable forms of behavior.

A second theoretical perspective underlying programs of this kind is the "total person" model of alcohol education. Its supporters criticize programs based primarily on the use of biological and pharmacological information, claiming that they ignore the social and psychological roots of deviant behavior. They contend that a shift is needed from simply disseminating information to the active involvement of participants in the solution of their problems. They assert that to reach the total person communication is vital, and that a tolerant, receptive atmosphere must be created in which ideas can be freely and honestly exchanged. They believe that the goal of alcoholism prevention programs should be to lead participants through a process of self-actualization, such that they will be able to function to their fullest potential, be guided by inner direction, and attain harmony between their internal beliefs and external actions. While its application in the school setting may be novel, this is not exactly a new idea. There is an ancient Hasidic saying: "The source of the difficulty between myself and other people is that too often I do not know what I feel, I do not say what I think, and I do not do what I say."

These programs stress the importance of the conformity phenomenon and peer group pressures. They attempt to prepare students emotionally for making behavioral choices on the basis of their own beliefs. In this light, they emphasize the importance of developing the courage to be different; honesty with oneself must be maintained, whether or not it assures popularity and peer approval. In short, programs of this type reflect the view that education must help youngsters develop a sense of responsibility and integrity in their human relations. To accomplish these goals they attempt to humanize education and focus on its social, emotional, and spiritual factors.

The main objective of affective education is to train youths to form activity groups within their schools, one of which would be involved in the development of alcohol education programs. The school programs may include experiences in affective processes, rap rooms, "people's problems" rooms, community problems classes, and alcohol education programs for younger children in elementary schools. A secondary goal is to train youths in group dynamics and communications techniques, such as values clarification, so that they can relate to other individuals on a similar affective level.

Effect of Primary Prevention Programs on Alcoholism

What impact have present-day alcohol education programs had on the reduction of alcoholism? "Very little, if any impact at all," concluded Donald Phelps, director of the division of prevention, National

Institute on Alcohol Abuse and Alcoholism, in an interview.[1] He further stated that it should be made clear to young people that "self-will is just as important as peer approval," and that "there should be no social stigma attached to the decision not to drink alcoholic beverages." He noted that the pressure on youths to drink usually comes from their peers. He further observed that "to be effective in alcoholism education, teachers need first to examine their own values; in dealing with alcoholism it is vital that we as teachers understand our own hang-ups before we begin dealing with the needs of students." In line with this personal opinion, data demonstrating the effectiveness of alcoholism prevention efforts are conspicuous by their absence.

Why have efforts of school districts to cope with the alcohol abuse problem had such disappointing effects? Several major limitations to their approaches can be identified on a *prima facie* basis. In the absence of a sound base of empirical data, this analysis necessarily reflects the personal observations of the authors.

First, most programs have focused attention on symptoms rather than on underlying factors that predispose individuals to use drugs, including alcohol. Many assume that if information is presented to students about the negative effects of alcohol, such information will tend to reduce its use. They completely ignore, however, factors such as the strains and pressures to which adolescents are exposed in their social relationships that may predispose them to use alcohol as a means of coping with these problems.

Second, these programs have generally been based on extremely simplistic models. They have not taken into account the fact that multiple and frequently conflicting social forces are simultaneously operating on young people. Alcohol programs introduced into schools that ignore the influence of both family and peer groups, for example, will have little probability of achieving their objectives.

Third, they have operated on the highly questionable assumption that the school and community environments in which alcohol programs are introduced can be ignored. They pay little attention to the fact that schools vary greatly in the extent to which students have trust and confidence in their teachers, health educators, and guidance officials and that neighborhoods and communities differ both in the social composition of their populations and in the consequent value orientation. To think that the same program will have similar effects when it is utilized in school and community environments that differ drastically is to operate, in our judgment, on a faulty assumption.

Fourth, and related to the above, little attention has been given to the possible necessity of developing *different* programs for student populations with different types of social and psychological needs. The assumption that a program that is meaningful and realistic for inner-city schools will also be effective for rural and suburban communities clearly needs to be challenged. Further, the same school system generally contains distinct sub-groups in the student population; this may necessitate the development of different strategies in influencing such different "target" populations.

Fifth, too few programs have recognized that effective programs require simultaneous focus on both fundamental psychological and social needs of young people and on the environment. For example, a program that attempts to provide arrangements whereby students can speak freely and openly about their fears and stresses but that ignores the external forces that create these problems cannot be expected to have any appreciable impact on the reduction of alcohol abuse.

Sixth, few programs have given consideration to the importance of the implementation phase of the new program. As noted earlier, this phase is critical in the change process, and to ignore it is to invite disaster. Teachers and health specialists require support from the school system and the community in introducing and carrying out an alcohol education program. Many educational professionals have either only a vague understanding of the central objectives of alcohol prevention programs or serious reservations about their utility. Many may require new skills. Moreover, other aspects of the operation of the school may need to be modified if the program is to succeed. These obstacles to the implementation of alcohol prevention programs have generally been ignored.

Seventh, few of these programs have given serious consideration to the importance of evaluation or to the necessity of building this component into the structure of the program. Unless evaluation is perceived as an integral part of the program, there will be no way to measure its efficacy.

Eighth, the designers of alcohol prevention programs have devoted a great deal of effort to their distribution but have seldom recognized that adaptation and flexibility may be required in new programs if they are to meet the needs of particular student populations. It is hardly conceivable that any single approach will prove to be universally valid.

Conclusion

It is our view that attempts in Pennsylvania at alcohol education and prevention have been largely unsuccessful. There are a multiplicity of reasons for this. Too many communities refuse to recognize the problem of alcohol abuse in their schools and feel that it is limited only to college level students and adults. Past attempts at alcohol abuse education in high schools have frequently been "one-shot" efforts which had little or no impact on attitudes. Educational materials and course outlines too often are outdated and not relevant to the current scene. Scare tactics are common. School districts frequently set punitive, unrealistic policies for handling problems of alcohol abuse within their jurisdiction. Teachers who have little or no rapport with the students and have received no guidance as to what to teach, how to teach, or when to teach are assigned to teach alcohol education courses. Frequently, the students know more about alcohol than do instructors. As a result of these misguided attempts, little success has been evidenced in preventive programs. In fact, it has been found that attitudes toward alcohol abuse become increasingly more positive as students traverse the grades in high school. This essentially means that current programs in alcohol abuse education have either had no effect or have succeeded in amplifying the positive attitudes which students already have about alcohol. At the very least, the programs have not been able to reverse the strong peer pressure for alcohol usage placed upon the student. In light of the tremendous impact of our educational system on young people and the obvious need for meaningful preventive alcohol abuse education programs, an expanded and innovative educational system is needed.

Our survey of this aspect of alcoholism, limited as it has been, has brought us to the belief that "the school must divorce itself from the traditional classroom concept and expand its frame of reference to make full use of all available community resources; museums, libraries, business and industry, and local government agencies all have a role to play in alcohol education."[2] Administrators and teachers should orchestrate these resources into a workable curriculum rather than concentrating exclusively on classroom materials. To accomplish this, it is imperative that a close working relationship be established among students, educators, businessmen, union leaders, and representatives of government at the local, regional, and state levels. This will assist in formulating educational programs and activities that are relevant to real life issues—and give students the values, attitudes, and methods they will need to solve present and future problems without resorting to alcohol. If the classroom is to prepare the student for the world, the boundary between the classroom and the world must become readily passable.

References

1. Phelps, D. Personal interview. Reported in NIAAA Newsletter, *Alcohol and Health Notes,* November 1973.

2. Barrett, M. The Pennsylvania state alcohol abuse and alcoholism plan for 1971-72, *Vol. 1: A design for action.* Harrisburg: Commonwealth of Pennsylvania, 1972, p. 126.

Section Four

CONCLUSIONS

Chapter 16

Summary of Findings

At the time the data were collected, the crucial findings of this study were as follows:

... there were 80 alcohol treatment programs in Pennsylvania.

... there were 6,805 alcoholics in treatment, representing about 1% of the total estimated number of alcoholics in the Commonwealth.

... white males comprised slightly over half of the treatment population.

... non-white males represented one-quarter of the alcoholics in treatment, but only 4% of the total population.

... in absolute numbers, non-white females had the lowest representation in treatment programs.

... the average age of the patients was 42.

... the most prevalent educational and occupational group was the high school educated blue collar worker.

... 44% of the patients were employed full-time, and 42% were receiving public assistance.

... 74 out of 80 program directors stated that their patients abused drugs other than alcohol, most commonly Librium®, Valium®, and barbiturates.

... patients treated in urban counties accounted for almost half of the alcoholics in treatment, Allegheny County with 27% and Philadelphia with 19%.

... the distribution of programs by counties tended to follow the distribution of the general population, except for Allegheny County, which had a greater proportion of programs than population and Philadelphia, having a smaller proportion of programs than population.

... counties dominated by small cities tended to be under-represented when patients in treatment are compared with the estimated number of persons in need of treatment; for every 149 alcoholics in the population of such counties there is only one in treatment as compared to a ratio of 139:1 for the entire state.

... urban programs tended to be larger than suburban, small town, and rural programs.

... of all patients in treatment, 95% were from Pennsylvania, and 80% received treatment in their county of residence.

... 23 out of 67 counties had no alcoholics in treatment.

... there is little relationship between the prevalence of alcoholism and the number of alcoholics in treatment in a county.

A classificatory system was devised in which programs were categorized by the function rather than the content of treatment. This was necessary since the nature of intervention offered was similar from program to program. Six functional components were identified. Existing programs consisted of either one of these components or of combinations of two or more components.

... more than 70% of all programs were comprised of only one component.

... no program contained all six components needed to provide comprehensive treatment.

... only one community had effective access to all components.

... over half of all patients were treated in single component programs.

... of all programs, 2.5% were of the five-component type; such programs treated 10% of all patients.

The distribution of components among single-component programs and among all programs was:

	Component	% of Single Component Programs	% of All Programs
I.	Acute Intervention (medical or non-medical)	3.5	15.1
II.	Evaluation (central diagnostic centre)	0.0	3.4
III.	Intensive Intervention (residential or day program)	15.8	19.3
IV.	Stabilization (halfway house)	17.5	14.3
V.	Maintenance (out-patient clinic)	61.4	44.5
VI.	Domiciliary care (some state hospitals)	1.8	3.4
		N = 57	N = 119

... there was a general lack of evaluation and domiciliary services.
... out-patient maintenance programs dominated the treatment effort, accounting for half of both the programs and patients.
... women were under-represented in halfway houses and comprehensive five-component programs.
... urban programs tended to have a high concentration of halfway houses and out-patient programs; treatment in rural areas is primarily out-patient maintenance.

Data collected on the staff of the 80 programs showed that:

... there was a total of 740 full-time and 365 part-time staff.
... the staffs were comprised of physicians (3%); mental health professionals (40%); recovered alcoholics (27.3%); and support personnel, such as secretaries and custodians (23%).
... almost one-quarter of the directors were physicians, almost one-half had graduate degrees, 10% had bachelor's degrees, 1% were ministers, and 9% had a high school education or less.
... out-patient maintenance clinics had the highest patient-to-staff ratio, 27:1, while detoxification and intensive in-patient programs had the lowest, 2:1 and 3:1, respectively, as compared to 9:1 for all programs.
... detoxification programs were dominated by professionally trained staff.
... intensive in-patient programs contained a large proportion of recovered alcoholics.

An informally conducted evaluation of the quality of the treatment programs yielded these results:

... three-quarters of the programs were judged to be of below-average quality.

... two-thirds of all patients were being treated in below-average programs.

... the most prevalent treatment component, out-patient maintenance, tended to receive the lowest-quality ratings.

... programs receiving high-quality ratings were generally comprised of four or more elements, had a high staff-to-patient ratio, were relatively small, and had recovered alcoholics on the treatment staff.

Information obtained about the directors' definitions of alcoholism, goals of treatment, and recommendations, indicated that:

... there was little correlation between program goals and program views on the nature of alcoholism.

... the medical disease concept and a combination of medical disease, psychological problems, and social functioning problems were the two most common definitions of alcoholism.

... abstinence and a combination of abstinence, alleviation of emotional problems, and improvement of social functioning were the two most common goals.

... three-quarters of the directors mentioned a need for particular types of treatment facilities in their communities, such as detoxification beds, halfway houses, and facilities of all sorts to meet the needs of female alcoholics.

... almost half recommended greater effort in the direction of education and prevention.

... over one-third expressed a need for more and better mechanisms for funding, and greater coordination between programs and between government and programs.

Information collected on the environment, both physical and social, in which the programs were operating yielded these results:

... there was a wide variety of facilities, ranging from an examining room in a hospital to an old farm house.

... almost half were located in hospitals, one-quarter in former private residences, and 12% in office buildings.

... non-urban facilities tended to be in better condition.

... few facilities were actually dilapidated, but most were unimaginative and drab.

... the relationship between the programs and the community was very positive.

... the relationship between the programs and the medical community was the least satisfactory of the relationships to those elements of the community which were examined. In particular, directors reported indifference and lack of cooperation on the part of private physicians and hospital emergency rooms.

In addition to the 80 programs which conformed to the stated criteria of an alcohol treatment program, two additional types of treatment enterprises were also included in the study. They are Alcoholics Anonymous and rescue missions, both of which have offered their services to alcoholics in Pennsylvania for many years. A small sample of the total number of these two types of service was visited. It was found that:

... the influence of AA was pervasive throughout the treatment system in Pennsylvania.
... two-thirds of the 80 treatment programs had at least one AA group associated with them, and at least half of the alcoholics who were patients in treatment programs were actively involved with AA as well.
... the population of alcoholics received by the rescue missions of the Salvation Army and the International Union of Gospel Missions is homogeneous—homeless men having little education, few job skills, and a long history of general social instability.
... the rescue missions are a permanent fixture on the skid rows of most American cities and provide services—at the very least, food, clothing, and shelter—to a population of alcoholics that is often unreached by other forms of treatment.

A number of efforts other than actual treatment exist in the Commonwealth in order to alleviate the problem of alcoholism. These are education and prevention programs, and industrial programs. A sample of each was visited, with these results:

... the number of alcoholics employed in industry in Pennsylvania is estimated to be 75,000.
... 15 companies throughout the Commonwealth have policies offering the alcoholic employee a chance to seek treatment while protecting his job.
... industrial programs can offer effective motivation to the alcoholic, and every effort should be made by the Commonwealth to aid employers in developing them.
... school and community education programs fall into four general types.
... they have been largely unsuccessful in deterring alcohol abuse.

From these disparate findings, the following conclusions have been drawn:

... no coherent, ongoing treatment system existed at the time of data collection.

... an aggregate of disjointed, largely entrepreneurial programs with little knowledge of one another comprised the treatment effort.

... the response on the local level to the problem of alcohol abuse was not guided by its prevalence, but rather by a variety of extraneous factors.

... therapeutic intervention was almost identical from program to program.

... most communities lacked convenient access to many or even most of the components necessary to comprehensive treatment.

... a follow-up study indicated that substantial overall increases in patients and decreases in staff were not the product of planned, deliberate changes but rather the result of random, sporadic shifts in individual programs.

... a permanent, ongoing reciprocal relationship between treatment and research is necessary, in the form of a uniform data collection system and readily available technical assistance.

... if consistently high quality care is to be effectuated, there must be a planned, systematic approach to the problem of alcoholism.

Chapter 17

Recommendations

System:
(1) A set or assemblage of things connected, associated, or interdependent, so as to form a complex unity; a whole composed of parts in orderly arrangement according to some scheme or plan; rarely applied to a simple or small assemblage of things (nearly = 'group' or 'set').

—Oxford English Dictionary,
vol.X, p.393

The foregoing 16 chapters of this book have presented a great deal of data on the treatment of alcoholism in Pennsylvania between December 1972 and December 1973. For the convenience of the reader these data have been summarized in the immediately preceding chapter. In the final chapter an attempt will be made to go beyond the data presented. The principal question to be addressed is: "What do the data mean in terms of a program of action for the future?"

While the authors will try to answer this question, any attempt to transcend empirical data is, by definition, speculative. One man's speculation may be another man's folly. Most data admit of alternative constructions, and it may not be possible to choose between the alternatives on purely objective grounds. There is no need to be apologetic for this; indeed, as is the case with works of art,[1] bodies of data may remain useful and relevant precisely because they are ambiguous and can be interpreted in different ways as conditions change and as knowledge advances. The major value of the present study lies in the material already presented. Nevertheless, it seems indicated at this point to provide an example of one possible interpretation, deriving from the perspective of those most familiar with the data and their limitations.

To summarize that interpretation at once: the data suggests that basic structural, qualitative, and quantitative changes need to be made in the approach to the treatment of alcoholism in Pennsylvania. The treatment of alcoholism needs to be systematized, broadened in scope, and increased in amount.

Structural Considerations: The Systemization of Treatment

That considerations of structure have been neglected in the development of alcoholism treatment should come as no surprise. Alcoholism treatment is a subdivision of the provision of health services, and health services in the United States have never been systematized. This very issue is currently of the greatest importance politically. A series of legislative measures beginning the process of systematization has been enacted by Congress; as a former Secretary of Health, Education, and Welfare has recently explained, the question is no longer whether this change will occur but merely when and in what form.[2]

Since at this writing the greater proportion of systematic change is still to come in health services generally, it is not unusual that it has not come in either alcoholism treatment or in other categorical treatment areas. A previous study[3] documented the lack of a systematic approach to the treatment of drug abuse in Pennsylvania. No evidence is immediately available which would suggest that a systematic approach is operating with respect to the treatment of other allied conditions, such as smoking, obesity, suicide, or home or motor vehicle accidents. The attempt to provide mental health services on a systematic basis through community mental health centres may represent the only major attempt at categorical treatment on a systematic basis, and even its staunchest proponents readily admit that it constitutes only a beginning. Hence the treatment of alcoholism is certainly not uniquely that sector of treatment which requires systematization.

The initial chapter of this book has also documented the fact that, historically, there never has been a comprehensive and rational approach to alcoholism treatment. A cognate chapter of the previous study demonstrated the same fact for narcotic addiction treatment; and of course it is also true for health care delivery as well. That is to say, our lack of a systematic approach in these fields is *not* the result of the breakdown of a prior system, but rather a direct continuation of the fact that there never has been a system. It is beyond the scope of the present work to go into the reasons for this in any detail. But it may be noted that a general lack of systematic treatment is to some extent a uniquely American phenomenon. The U.S. is the only major industrialized country in the world without a national health system. Our antipathy to systems in the health sphere seems in some important respects to mirror our antipathy to systems in the economic sphere. This in turn may be traced directly to the thinking of Dr. Adam Smith, an 18th century Scotsman. He believed that the (hopefully) enlightened self-interest of individuals operating in the economic sphere would automatically result in the greatest good for the greatest number. That this doctrine should appear increasingly inadequate as we approach the 21st century does not reflect undue discredit upon Dr. Smith. Times have changed, and few doctrines can withstand the accumulated weight of three centuries of human experience. Whether a systematic approach to economics was needed or not in Dr. Smith's day will not be argued. But the major recommendation of this study is that systematization of the alcoholism treatment effort in Pennsylvania is needed now.

To highlight some of the evidence that this is the case, such facts as the imbalance of the current treatment effort may be cited. Chapter 4 documents that, from a programmatic viewpoint, the treatment system is completely dominated by the out-patient clinic, which comprises more than 60% of all of the single component programs and occurs in more than half of all programs taken together, far in excess of any other component (Table 5). This most dominant program component was also of singularly low quality; only 16.7% were rated "good" (see Chapter 10). Conversely, those programs which received the best quality ratings, the multi-component programs with a branched structure, were relatively rare. There also seemed to be a palpable lack of some of the other critical treatment components, such as diagnostic and domiciliary facilities, and to a lesser extent halfway houses and acute care units. Chapter 9 suggests that these lacunae are apparent to treatment program directors.

These are structural considerations. Evidence that the current programs do not *function* as a system is apparent from Chapter 11, in which changes in programs were measured over time. It was obvious that the changes which occurred were random and erratic, and were guided by no rational principles. Some further evidence may be derived from data in Chapter 5, which indicated that there was no relationship, on a county-by-county basis, between the prevalence of alcoholism and the availability of treatment for alcoholism. Since most patients (80%) seek treatment in their own county, this is a more important finding than the supposed mobility of the population might suggest. To this evidence may be added the impressions of survey staff that programs did not relate to each other in any regular manner. Frequently, they were unaware of the nature or (rarely) even of the existence of other programs. No evidence of cross-referral to any significant degree was apparent, even in many of the single component programs. As will be noted from the definition at the head of this chapter, *relationship* is the essential ingredient of a systematic approach. Alcoholism treatment programs were *not* found to be "connected, associated, or interdependent." An alcoholism treatment system did not exist.

As has already been noted, alcoholism treatment is not alone in being unsystematic. Nor is alcoholism treatment in Pennsylvania unique. Workers in Alaska[4] and in the state of Washington[5,6] have documented the same phenomenon. Based on their experience in North Carolina, a team of investigators made the following eloquent statement:

> *Historically the public response to the alcoholic or problem drinker or to the collective problem called "alcoholism" has been partial and segmented.... To view this situation through "systems eyes" reveals a cluttered, disjointed, overlapping, uncoordinated, and ineffective set of public and private programs that are opportunistic and responsive primarily to an immediate crisis or community tension. Lacking is a purposeful and continuing system that approaches the problem both at the micro (individual drinker) and macro (community) levels, that is able to bring together current resources and activities effectively, and that is responsive to changes in the population served.*[7]

Based upon the experience of the survey team in Pennsylvania and of other investigators elsewhere, therefore, it is the principal recommendation of this study that all necessary steps be taken to systematize the treatment of alcoholism in Pennsylvania. It remains to be specified just how this might be accomplished. Because it is an unfortunate fact of history that severe and autocratic measures may be taken in the name of system establishment, it should be said at once that the establishment of a treatment system does *not* involve the destruction of existing treatment programs. On the contrary, if, as we shall suggest below, the total effort in the treatment area is quantitatively inadequate, such a course would be disastrous. At the present time, the Commonwealth needs every bit of treatment activity it can muster in the field of alcoholism, and more.

To employ a simple analogy which has been useful previously,[8] let us follow the steps that might be taken by a heating engineer who was called upon to put together a heating system. He might first visit the construction site to assess the raw materials provided for the system by the contractor. The assessment would be both qualitative and quantitative, and as a result he would know how much of what materials he had on hand, and how adequate they were. As a result of this first phase of his work he would probably find that some of his materials were of inadequate quality and that other essential ingredients were missing. Hence he would set about to improve the quality of what he had on hand and would ask the contractor to provide whatever was missing. He might mend some of the equipment, might put a new door on the furnace here or bore out a pipe there; and he might order some new valves which were required. Finally, when he had all the equipment he needed, and it was of sufficient adequacy, he would connect it so that it would work. Pipes, valves, furnace, and radiators would all be assembled in an appropriate functional relationship to one another. Finally, he would stoke up the furnace and see whether the system, working in an integrated manner, would deliver an adequate and controlled amount of heat to the rooms of the house.

By analogy, the present study, at the time it was done, was similar to the first action of assessment by the heating engineer. However, as Chapter 11 indicates, treatment programs are dynamic phenomena. They change over time. Hence what is required is a *continuous* monitoring of the status of the components of the treatment system. One-shot studies will not adequately describe an entity which is continually in a state of flux. To some extent, description on a continuing, longitudinal basis can be subserved by such instruments as the Uniform Data Collection System, which should provide basic data on every program at stated periods.

Whether it will be possible for such a data collection system to serve more than as an indicator of the vicissitudes of program quality is, however, debatable. Beyond this, there is the related problem of providing the necessary input to improve program quality. Chapter 10 amply documents that efforts at the improvement of quality are essential at least concurrently with, and probably prior to, the assembly of a functional system. A system is only as strong as its weakest component, and there is little sense in constructing one that consists largely of sub-standard elements. Our study suggests strongly that certain factors may be related to program quality, such as staff-patient ratios, and holds out the promise that if these factors were more systematically identified they could be applied across the entire group of programs to good effect. But it seems inescapable that the mounting of such an ambitious program will require human input and cannot simply be done on paper. Constant program monitoring by informed, sympathetic, effective, and enlightened individuals will probably turn out to be a *sine qua non* for the development of an effective treatment system. Hopefully the interlocking systems of regional offices and single county authorities can be developed to fill these needs.

Assuming that existing components can be brought up to and/or maintained at an adequate level of quality, there remains the question of the design of the functional system which will relate the parts "so as to form a complex unity." In attempting to categorize the components of treatment (Chapter 4) a simple functional diagram was developed. This diagram outlined what appeared to be a logical inter-relationship between existing components in the field, and one which, moreover, actually held in those few programs having multiple components. What will be proposed here is a further modification of this basic structure. It resembles the core-shell treatment model system which has been suggested[9,10] as being useful in the treatment of drug abuse (Figure 1).

The essential feature of this model is that it limits access to definitive treatment by structurally requiring the exercise of differential diagnostic procedures for each episode of care. No patient would gain initial access to treatment through a definitive treatment program (in the terminology of this report, components III, IV or VI, that is, intensive intervention, stabilization, or domiciliary care). Patients entering a new episode of treatment from the community would first pass through a diagnostic process (in some instances after acute intervention had occurred) designed to assess their unique treatment needs. On the basis of this assessment they would be assigned to that treatment program most likely to produce a positive result. If this did not "take," they would be sent back to the diagnostic unit for re-evaluation and reassignment, with a presumption that a satisfactory "match" between patient and treatment program could be found. In other words, the structure of this treatment system would provide *for every patient* the possibility of more than a single definitive treatment option—the kind of branched-chain schematic design found only in a small number of current treatment programs and associated also with high program quality.

Behind the assumption that alternative plans of treatment are desirable is the assumption that the population of persons who suffer from problems related to alcohol is a heterogeneous population that will not respond in the same manner to the same kinds of treatment. Many people with long clinical experience in the field of alcoholism have intuitively recognized that this is indeed the case and that, for example, the corporation executive whose productive life is complicated by alcohol is rather different in terms of the kinds of treatment he requires than the long-term habitue of skid row who may never in his lifetime have achieved the former patient's level of social competence. It must be admitted that others with equally lengthy clinical experience will controvert this. But the research evidence seems to substantiate the essential heterogeneity of alcoholic populations, at least as they present themselves for treatment. For example, when all admissions to four different treatment facilities in the state of Washington over a two-month period were intensively assessed with a variety of instruments, significant differences between all four populations could be documented.[11] In Alaska, definite differences between patients as to the staging of the seriousness of their

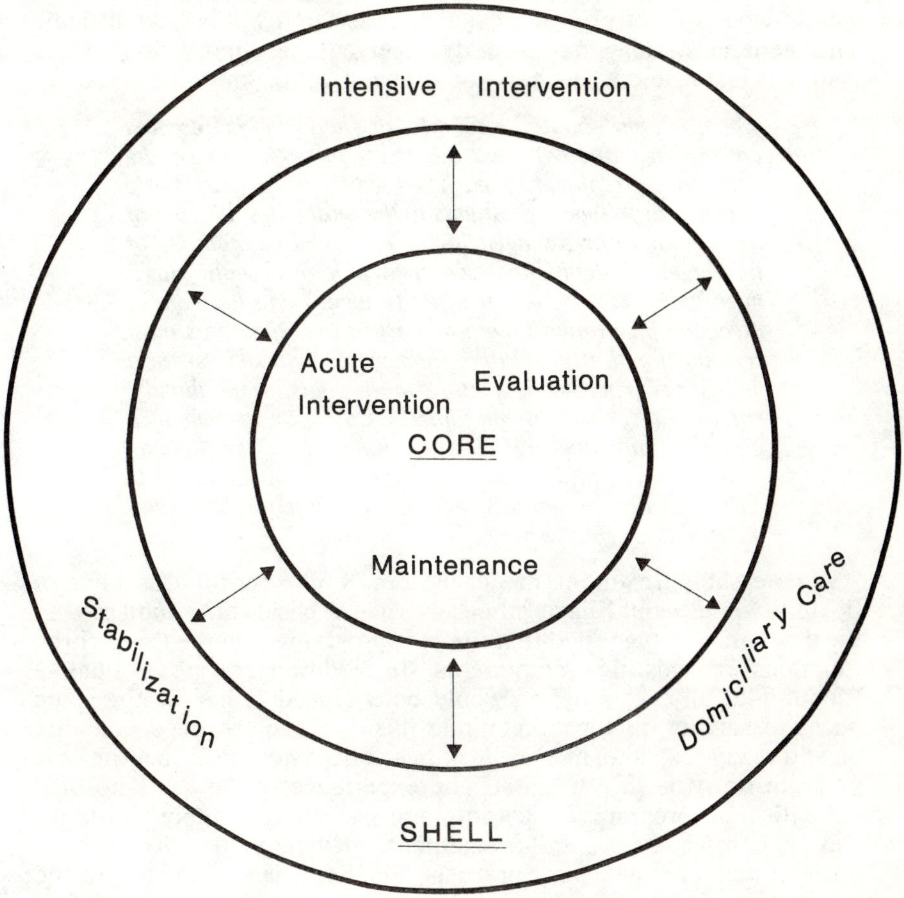

Figure 1 —The Core-Shell Treatment System Model for Alcoholism impairment could be shown.[12] If the population is indeed heterogeneous, and if truly different treatment paradigms are available, the possibility is raised that the scrupulous matching of individuals to treatment programs will improve clinical results. In addition, of course, if something can be done to sharpen the ability to discern who will do well in what kind of program, evaluative research will be less difficult. This general strategy has recently received the approbation of the National Institute on Alcohol Abuse and Alcoholism:

> *... programs should take into account the differences among the patients...and systematically seek to fit the appropriate treatment to each individual...it is possible to match certain types of patients to the most suitable types of helping facilities or agencies or programs or methods of treatment. Undoubtedly, treatment programs could maximize their effectiveness by clearly identifying the type of alcoholic population they propose to serve, the goals most feasible for that population, and what methods can most nearly be expected to achieve those goals. Undoubtedly, success rates could be maximized if the expectations of a group of patients are sensibly matched to the helping resource. And, in this context, it would become possible to carry out tightly designed evaluations that would clearly measure the effectiveness of each program.*[13]

A core-shell treatment model system would permit this kind of flexibility, and would have other advantages besides. As indicated in the diagram, it is suggested that the core program subsume three of the functions of existing components. In addition to the evaluative function, a full core program would be equipped to handle the acute phase of alcohol intoxication. While this does require the availability of, and ready access to, medical facilities, it does not mean that the core program must be in a hospital. The experience of the extra-hospital detoxification programs in Toronto and elsewhere[14] amply substantiates that this is a feasible arrangement. In view of the high cost of hospital beds it is also very practical. Finally, it is suggested that the core program be equipped to provide the maintenance function of an out-patient clinic.

One of the principal advantages of such an arrangement is that it is readily exportable to any location in the state. It is believed that any jurisdiction would be able to support and staff a core program. Virtually all of the functions which a core program would be called upon to exercise can be and historically have been performed by ancillary personnel under the supervision of trained professionals. Most out-patient clinics and detoxification centres are currently operated in this manner. Differential diagnosis can be systemized into an instrument which can be effectively utilized by appropriately trained individuals from diverse backgrounds, as has happened with a similar diagnostic instrument in the drug abuse field.[15] Some will argue that the intensive use of non-professionals will militate against a high quality of program, but the evidence gathered in this study suggests the opposite. Hence it seems within the realm of possibility that even the more remote areas of the Commonwealth could support a core program. This would permit in most cases the greatest part of the patient's time to be spent in his community, a highly desirable feature as well.

There is another advantage. The definitive treatment programs in the alcoholism field seem to have become identified in the public mind with end-stage alcoholism. As will be argued below, there is some validity to this association. The new core programs could be presented to the public in a different light, principally as evaluation centres, though with the capability of handling much more than evaluation should that be necessary. The core program could handle, quite by itself, those less severe problems related to alcohol which do not require residential treatment of any kind. Hence it might very well happen that those persons with lesser degrees of involvement in alcohol-related problems than end-stage alcoholism will feel more congenial about entering treatment, as their entrance will not necessarily identify them as alcoholics—which by most definitions of that word they are not.

In contrast to the core programs, the shell programs would subserve a variety of definitive and for the most part residential interventions. They constitute the costly element of treatment. For this reason there is every hope that a given shell facility would be utilized by more than one core program. Such facilities ought to be treated as statewide, rather than merely local, resources. It is unlikely that there will ever be enough of them to permit the luxury of a single core program affiliation. The important thing is that every shell facility be related to a core program, and that every core program have access to at least one of each kind of shell facility. This fulfills the requirements of the model, and at the same time conserves resources.

One of the most important features of such an arrangement is the facilitatory effect it would have upon information flow, and upon research based on information. At present, and in the past, one of two strategies has usually been adopted to obtain crucial baseline data on patients entering treatment. Either an independent research team has been hired to perform this function, or the clinical personnel at the program level have been asked (or more commonly, ordered) to do it. The former approach is too expensive and the latter too disruptive and almost always inaccurate. Program personnel are interested in treatment, not in research. Administrative fiat will not alter this, as it is based on a fundamental difference in approach; research questions everything, while treatment demands the acceptance of a certain set of basic assumptive beliefs as inviolable. Convert a therapist into a researcher and you will likely erode his therapeutic efficacy. One of the major advantages of the core program - shell program arrangement is that the heaviest data collection tasks fall upon core program personnel who at most are involved in the less demanding treatment requirements of a maintenance program. The data demands on definitive intervention personnel, while there will be some, will be much less; in particular, the extensive baseline data will already have been gathered by the time the patient arrives at the definitive treatment program.

Given that this data can be thus efficiently gathered, it permits a much more ready approach to research. On account of the limited access to definitive intervention, cohorts of patients for follow-up studies can be selected from successive admissions to the core program, rather than to the definitive treatment program as is now the case. This is important because, as is suggested above, a given patient may be tried in more than one kind of definitive treatment in order to receive the optimum result. The fundamental question in follow-up studies when approached from a systems perspective is *not* whether a *given* program is effective. It is rather whether a given *patient* can extract from the universe of treatment possibilities available to him all the kinds of intervention which are necessary in whatever order and in whatever amount to produce a result which satisfactorily meets his or her unique treatment needs. Any program which can *contribute* to this result for a particular population of patients is a justifiable program. It is not necessary, as has been implied by previous follow-up study design, that a given program must show that it and it alone can produce highly effective results in an unselected sample of cases. The pessimism which currently surrounds treatment stems in large measure from such unrealistic expectations.

Moreover, it must be recognized that neither the patient population nor the modes of intervention being exercised are static. They all change. They are not the same today as they were yesterday. Anyone with clinical experience recognizes that treatment programs evolve, that their thrust depends upon transient qualities, that a few staff who may come or go may make a profound difference in the program's overall impact. By selecting serial cohorts from the core program, following them up, and correlating outcomes with interventions, a continuous feedback of data can be created with which in turn the referral process can be repeatedly restructured. If it is found on one occasion that a particular type of patient does well in a particular program, it cannot be assumed that this will be so for an infinite period of time. Perhaps next year the same kind of patient will do better in another program (or in another set of programs or another sequence of programs). By following up serial cohorts of admissions to the core program this can be observed and the referral process can be adjusted accordingly. The North Carolina researchers found a happy metaphor to distinguish this type of dynamic approach from the usual static conceptualization:

A simplistic comparison. . .is between the technologically sophisticated heat-seeking missile and the torpedo. The former is constructed to collect and process information—in this case signals of heat intensity—in order to continuously change its flight course in seeking its target, a maneuvering jet aircraft; the latter, once launched, cannot change its course no matter what changes occur in the target.[16]

Similar results might conceivably be achieved by developing more programs which contain a complete range of components within them, rather than having core programs and different shell programs under separate auspices. While this is preferable to the current situation of program *anomie* and already exists to a small extent, there are suggestions[17,18] that this might be a less attractive alternative. Programs which are under uniform auspices tend to develop a uniform outlook. They grow to resemble each other in their basic assumptions and hence provide less in the way of alternative treatment strategies than might otherwise be the case. It may be preferable to permit definitive treatment to be a matter of different church, rather than a matter of same church, different pew. Strongly-held belief systems tend to be evangelical and will spread if under uniform auspices. As many programs in the field derive ultimately from religious sources, the analogy is not as farfetched as it may seem.[19] A major advantage of the core-shell treatment system model may be that it permits the incorporation of diverse functioning elements into a dynamic whole without compromising that individuality of approach which is the creative essence of therapeutic intervention.

Having suggested the systematization of alcoholism treatment and outlined how it might be accomplished, it is now necessary to post a major *caveat.* While it is a reasonable assumption that systematic treatment of the type envisioned would produce superior results to the non-systematic treatment which the study suggests usually obtains, it is only an assumption. The superiority of systematic treatment, at least in this field, has not been conclusively demonstrated.

Therefore, to move precipitously into such an approach on a large scale would be premature. Such a difficult and costly effort should have the benefit of a much more precise pilot evaluation prior to its widespread implementation. This ought to include, at minimum, a very carefully designed experimental test of the efficacy of systematic versus nonsystematic intervention. The experiment ought to be designed to determine not only whether systematic treatment is superior but to what degree and at what cost. In order to justify such a profound change, systematic treatment would have to be shown to be a great deal more effective and a great deal less costly.

However certain one may be that this will prove to be the case, those responsible for the disbursement of public funds must necessarily await the development of such data. With it, they can move ahead with confidence and, indeed, will stand a far better chance of obtaining whole-hearted cooperation with their efforts, both from those involved directly in intervention and from the general public. Without it, a natural resistance to change from accustomed procedures to new but unproven ones and a reluctance to underwrite the start-up costs for such a venture are only to be expected.

Qualitative Considerations: The Diversification of Treatment

One of the most striking findings of this study was that the treatment being provided in different programs in Pennsylvania was essentially the same kind of treatment. It did not vary. If different treatments were like different colors, treatment in Pennsylvania could be described as monochromatic. This was, to be sure, an impressionistic finding, and the survey team did not utilize an objective measure which could discriminately characterize intervention.[20] Such a complex procedure would have been well beyond the scope of the present research. But it was a sufficiently strong impression that it forced a restructuring of the taxonomic system used to classify treatment programs, a task which was not lightly undertaken. For a further description of this process and a characterization of treatment intervention as it was viewed by the survey team, the reader is referred to Chapter 4.

If a reason for this state of affairs is to be found in the data, it is probably imbedded in Table 3 of Chapter 3, which cross-tabulates program definitions of alcoholism with program goals. While there was a general lack of congruence between the two, it was also noted that "when alcoholism was defined solely in terms of the disease concept, 80% of the responses fell into the category either of abstinence or a combination of abstinence and one or more other goals . . . it seems that the disease concept, or some variation of it, is pervasive in the treatment field. The same is true for its treatment implication, abstinence (p.16). Chapter 13, dealing with Alcoholics Anonymous, further extends this conclusion by documenting that the association between treatment programs and AA was very close. Two-thirds of all programs had at least one AA group associated with them, and at least half of the alcoholics who were patients in treatment programs were actively involved in AA as well. Finally, Chapter 6 documents that almost 30% of the staff of these programs were ex-alcoholics, virtually all of them AA graduates.

Hence it would seem that the uniformity of treatment being provided in Pennsylvania at the time of the survey was largely the result of the dominant position of Alcoholics Anonymous and its conceptualizations within the treatment system. It should be said at once that this does not imply any criticism of AA. On the contrary, it is a tribute to the historical role of the organization. For 40 years it has borne the primary responsibility for treatment and has put the record of the helping professions in this area to shame. Our debt to AA can never be estimated, let alone settled. It remains a viable and important resource, as Chapter 13 abundantly documents. If a new interest in treatment intervention in alcoholism has had as one of its results the development of alternative concepts and strategies, AA may in large measure take credit for having stimulated these recent developments.

It is now time for others to step forward and to share with AA the burden that it has shouldered so well for so long. In particular, the dominance of the disease concept and of total abstinence as the only feasible treatment goal must be abated. It must be seen in perspective, a perspective undistorted by the great vacuum which hitherto existed in the treatment field and which the disease-abstinence model rushed in to fill. Scholars may question the validity of the disease model in an absolute sense.[21,22] But in terms of the treatment system this is not necessary. Past experience has amply demonstrated that, irrespective of its objective validity, the medical model of alcoholism has proven congenial to many therapists and to many patients. Extirpating it would be grotesque and is not required, since the proposed treatment system model can readily incorporate diverse viewpoints. What is required, however, is that a period of co-existence with alternative models now begin. This will require that the overzealous among the AA membership, who view its way as the only way to think about alcoholism and abstinence as the only treatment, may need to back off. They must recognize that theirs is an effective treatment and an heuristic model for many afflicted individuals—and that for others, alternatives may exist. That this is not too much to ask has been amply illustrated in the course of this study through discussion with many AA members.

The necessity of this possibly painful step relates to the effects which the dominance of one model may have on the treatment system. In addition to making treatment uniform, it tends to define the population of patients upon whom that treatment is to be exercised. It was the observation of the survey team that by far the greatest portion of the overall treatment effort in Pennsylvania was directed toward a single type of alcoholic: the chronic public inebriate, the end stage alcoholic. It is certainly true that such individuals require help, and also that they are not receiving it to the degree that is required (see below). But there are other kinds of people who have problems related to alcohol who are *not* currently receiving help. This is largely because of the skewing of the overall treatment effort toward the chronic public inebriate. This skewing, in turn, seems a direct result of the dominance of the medical-abstinence model, and of its corollary that an alcoholic must hit bottom before recovery is possible. This defines people as unsuitable objects for intervention until such time as they have hit bottom, and therein lie serious difficulties.

TABLE I

Percentage of patients by age range in alcoholism and drug abuse treatment programs, Philadelphia, Pennsylvania, October 1973 - March 1974 inclusive. Calculated from *Point Prevalence Study of Philadelphia Treatment Programs,* unpublished data of the Section on Drug and Alcohol Abuse.

Age Range	% of Patients, Alcoholism Treatment Programs	% of Patients, Drug Abuse Treatment Programs
Thru age 15	0.0	1.1
16 - 20	0.9	13.2
21 - 25	4.7	33.8
26 - 30	9.4	22.4
31 - 40	29.4	17.9
41 - 50	31.2	9.2
51 - 99	24.4	2.4
	100.0	100.0

$X^2 = 306.82$, p. exceeds .0005

Careful studies of a national household sample[24] have shown that the age incidence of problems related to alcoholism is highest during the 20s. The present study has found that the average age of patients in treatment in Pennsylvania is 42. It suggests that, on the average, a Pennsylvanian must experience problems related to alcohol for 20 years or more before receiving help. This is unacceptable. Surely intervention of some kind must be mounted without waiting for more than two decades. In the cognate field of drug abuse, treatment at an early age is the rule rather than the exception, in contrast to the field of alcoholism (Table 1). There is no reason to think that this could not be changed. The two problems are similar, both in time of onset and in nature. The difference of age distribution of patients in treatment, which is highly significant, appears to be due to beliefs about who is a proper candidate for treatment. These ideas, including the notion that an alcoholic must "hit bottom" prior to successful treatment, are socially rather than scientifically determined. Hence a strenuous attempt must be launched to provide treatment for that population which has the highest incidence of alcohol-related problems—the young. This is a serious deficiency in the Commonwealth. It is not limited to Pennsylvania, but has been seen as a problem of national importance.[24]

Nor are the young the only sub-population with problems related to alcohol who are not being adequately helped. There is evidence in this study that there may be a need for additional programs for women, and especially for black women. With respect to black men, it is interesting that in spite of their over-representation in the treatment system, there are few black AA groups. Perhaps some equivalent is needed. Other groups not addressed by this study, such as the aged, the Indians, and others, may all require the development of particular approaches.

The overall point is that the spectrum of kinds of treatment intervention for alcohol-related problems in Pennsylvania must be broadened. It must become polychromatic. It must match in its complexity and variety the complexity and variety of the problem. A part of the difficulty, to be sure, is the lack of alternative models to the medical model; but alternatives do exist.[25] Many may not be attractive. Others, such as the behavioral models, are beyond question attractive to many and have been applied widely outside of Pennsylvania. Indeed, with its lack of emphasis upon either the disease concept as an explanatory device or abstinence as the end result of intervention, the behavioral model of alcoholism may appeal to just those populations which are "turned off" by the medical model. There is no reason why an intelligently-designed treatment system could not incorporate within itself, from a functional point of view, these antithetical approaches, assigning to each those patients who would be likely to find them most congenial. In like manner it is hoped that a sufficient variety of models and resultant programs will eventually come to be included, so that effective and compatible treatment may be offered to the many disparate sub-populations who require it.

Quantitative Considerations: The Enlargement of Treatment

All of the foregoing discussion implies what everyone knows to be true: that there is not a sufficient amount of treatment for alcoholism available in Pennsylvania at the present time. Table IV of Chapter 1 indicates that fewer than one in every 100 abusers of alcohol could find a treatment slot available for him in the Commonwealth. While one may call for increasingly refined estimates of incidence, prevalence, and the number of treatment slots, the likelihood is that this proportion will not be significantly altered. Moreover, in certain areas of the Commonwealth, and particularly in those countries dominated by small cities (e.g., Bucks, Berks, Lehigh, Lancaster, Westmoreland, and others), there existed fewer than one treatment slot for every *200* alcohol abusers. It is cold comfort to find that Pennsylvania shares this problem as well with the nation at large. One of the principal findings of a recent survey by the federal government was that

> *Although the accessibility and quality of alcoholism treatment services are improving, there remains a serious deficit of such services, and only a small portion of alcoholic people are receiving the services required.*

Moreover, the bulk of treatment services which are available are designed to respond to late-stage alcoholism and do not meet the needs of people whose alcoholism is identified at earlier stages of the illness.[26]

There is reason to believe that the situation may become even more serious. More Americans are drinking alcoholic beverages, and this is especially true among the young.[27] If the proposed changes in the treatment system occur, they may have the effect of making treatment more acceptable, and a greater percentage of individuals with problems related to alcohol will seek treatment. Diversion of alcoholics from the criminal justice system, while humane, will markedly increase the demand for treatment if practised on a large scale. Third party coverage of alcohol-related problems is an increasing trend and may become a part of a national health insurance plan, thus eliminating financial barriers to treatment and presumptively also increasing demand. On the other hand the current economic situation is diminishing government revenues, while at the same time there is a general movement toward a reduction of government spending, particularly in the human services area. These are among the several factors which will tend to increase the discrepancy between the demand for treatment and its availability in the immediate future.

It is therefore obligatory to press for a significant expansion of treatment capability. At the same time, however, the fact must be faced that the expansion of treatment to cover even those who *wish* to be treated, let alone those who *need* to be treated, is most probably a manifest impossibility. Even if the will were there, the fiscal resources would not be. And this is not to mention the pool of skilled manpower that would be needed. It is a dilemma which is as true of the health field generally as it is of the field of alcoholism treatment. The government of Canada, for example, which for the last two decades has instituted most of the alterations in the health system referred to above, has found itself unable to continue the expansion of the system to meet an ever-increasing demand. "Since direct health care is already consuming some 7% of the wealth that Canadians produce annually," the minister of National Health and Welfare noted in a government working paper, "it is evident that the rate at which the government of Canada can expand its activities in the field of health is severely limited by financial considerations.[28]

This is not to say that government should not proceed with plans to rationalize, improve, and expand the treatment system, whether with respect to alcoholism or health generally. That it must do so is the major recommendation of this report. But it is also obligatory to recognize that this will not suffice to improve the overall health picture of the population. Treatment never does. No known disease has ever succumbed to effective treatment *as a disease,* though individual cases have been successfully treated. In like manner the treatment of alcoholism will be highly successful in many cases, but it will not substantially alter the problem of alcoholism for society. This would be true even if the financial limitations referred to did not exist.

The inescapable conclusion is that if there is to be any parity between the *need* for alcoholism treatment services and the *availability* of those services, it will come about not through a massive expansion of services but through a reduction in the need for them.[29] The only effective means for dealing with the problem of alcoholism will ultimately be to prevent it from occurring in the first place. This is a reality which must be faced. Other governments have done so:

> *Until now most of society's efforts to improve health, and the bulk of direct health expenditures, have been focused on the health care organization. Yet, when we identify the present main causes of sickness and death in Canada, we find that they are rooted in the other three elements of the [health field] concept: human biology, environment, and lifestyle. It is apparent, therefore, that vast sums are being spent treating diseases that could have been prevented in the first place. Greater attention to the first three conceptual elements is needed if we are to continue to reduce disability and early death.*[30]

It is not a pretty prospect. We do not know a great deal about the modification of a meretricious lifestyle such as alcoholism in the direction of increased health; about what Griffith Edwards refers to as "this peculiar business of edging people into changing their behaviour."[31] We had better learn. There does not seem to be any alternative. Some promising leads are available. As Edwards himself suggests, a generic approach to prevention may be helpful. We may learn much from researches in fields other than alcoholism, such as suicide prevention and the prevention of crime, of smoking, and of accidents. Superlative research by the staff of the Addiction Research Foundation in Toronto has suggested that there may be measures which the government could take which would be effective in the reduction of alcoholism, or would at least contain it at its current levels (see Appendix D).[32] But there is little question that much work as well as much soul-searching lies ahead.

Given all of this, we are finally faced with a paradox. Given the weight of our past record and of our present ignorance, how can we afford to have hope for the future? Given the immediacy of our current needs, how can we afford not to have hope?

References

1. Kris, E. *Psychoanalytic explorations in art.* New York: International Universities Press, 1952.

2. Richardson, E.L. "The old order changeth, yielding place to new": perspectives on the health revolution. *New England Journal of Medicine,* Aug. 8, 1974, *291:* 283-87.

3. Adler, F., Moffett, A.D., Glaser, F.B., et al. *A systems approach to drug treatment.* Philadelphia: Dorrance & Co., 1975.

4. Miller, S., Helmick, E., Berg, L., et al. Alcoholism: A statewide program evaluation. *American Journal of Psychiatry.* Feb. 1974, *131:* 210-14.

5. Pattison, E.M., Coe, R., and Rhodes, R.J. Evaluation of alcoholism treatment: A comparison of three facilities. *Archives of General Psychiatry,* April 1969, *20:* 478-88.

6. Pattison, E.M., Coe, R., and Doerr, H.O. Population variation among alcoholism treatment facilities. *International Journal of the Addictions,* 1973, *8,* 199-229.

7. Holder, H.D. and Stratas, N.E. A systems approach to alcoholism programming. *American Journal of Psychiatry.* July 1972, *129:* 32-37.

8. Adler, et al., *op.cit.*

9. *Ibid.*

10. Glaser, F.B. The treatment of drug abuse in the rural South: Application of the core-shell treatment system model. *Southern Medical Journal,* May 1974, *67:* 580-86. Abstracted in *Rural and Community Medicine,* December 1974, *81:* 32.

11. Pattison, Coe, & Doerr, *op.cit.*

12. Miller, et al., *op.cit.*

13. Chafetz, M.E. and Keller, M. (ed.). *Alcohol and health: New knowledge.* DHEW Publication No. (ADM) 74-124. Washington, D.C.: Government Printing Office, 1974 (Preprint Edition), p.145.

14. O'Briant, R.G., Lennard, H.L., Allen, S.D., et al. *Recovery from alcoholism: A social treatment model.* Springfield: Charles C. Thomas, 1973.

15. Pittel, S.M. and Hofer, R. A systematic approach to drug treatment referral. *Journal of Psychedelic Drugs,* April-June 1974, *6:* 253-58.

16. Holder & Stratas, *op.cit.*, p.33.

17. Pattison, Coe & Rhodes, *op.cit.*

18. Pattison, Coe & Doerr, *op.cit.*

19. Glaser, F.B. Some historical aspects of the drug-free therapeutic community. *American Journal of Drug & Alcohol Abuse,* May 1974, *1:* 37-52.

20. Moos, R. *Revision of the ward atmosphere scales: Technical report.* Stanford, California: Social Ecology Laboratory, Department of Psychiatry, Stanford University, 1971.

21. Edwards, G. The status of alcoholism as a disease. *In: Modern trends in drug dependence and alcoholism,* ed. R.V. Phillipson. New York: Appleton-Century-Crofts, 1970, pp.140-163.

22. Robinson, D. The alcohologist's addiction: Some implications of having lost control over the disease concept of alcoholsim. *Journal of Studies on Alcohol,* Dec. 1972, 33: 1028-59.

23. Cahalan, D. *Problem drinkers.* San Francisco: Jossey-Bass, 1970.

24. Chafetz and Keller, *op.cit.,* p.146.

25. Siegler, M., Osmond, H., and Newell, S. Models of alcoholism. *Journal of Studies on Alcohol.* Sept. 1968, *29:* 571-91.

26. Chafetz & Keller, *op.cit.,* p.xii.

27. *Ibid.,* pp.8-12.

28. Lalonde, M. *A new perspective on the health of Canadians: A working document.* Ottawa: Government of Canada, April 1974, p. 65.

29. Somers, A.R. Recharting national health priorities: A new Canadian perspective. *New England Journal of Medicine,* (Aug. 22) 1974, *291:* 415-16.

30. Lalonde, *op.cit.,* p.32.

31. Edwards, G. Alternative strategies for minimizing alcohol problems: Coming out of the doldrums. Manuscript. Presented at the Expert Conference on the Prevention of Alcohol Problems, Berkeley, California, December 9-11, 1974, p.26.

32. Addiction Research Foundation. Proposal for a Comprehensive Health-Oriented Alcohol Control Policy in Ontario. Mimeographed. Toronto, April 1973.

Appendix A

TABLES

TABLE A-1

Number of Alcohol Programs and Alcohol Patients in Treatment, By County

County Population			Programs		Alcoholics in Treatment	
County	1970 Pop.	%	No.	%	No.	%
Category I	3,553,625	30.1	24	30.0	3127	46.0
Allegheny	1,605,016	13.6	17	21.2	1831	26.9
Philadelphia	1,948,609	16.5	7	8.8	1296	19.0
Category II	1,223,834	10.3	9	11.3	742	10.9
Delaware	600,035	5.1	4	5.0	443	6.5
Montgomery	623,799	5.2	5	6.3	299	4.4
Category III	3,889,873	32.8	24	30.0	1582	23.4
Adams	56,937	0.5	—	—	—	—
Berks	296,382	2.5	2	2.5	176	2.6
Bucks	415,471	3.5	2	2.5	46	0.7
Chester	278,311	2.4	4	5.0	222	3.3
Dauphin	233,834	2.0	3	3.7	46	0.7
Erie	263,654	2.2	2	2.5	107	1.6
Greene	36,090	0.3	—	—	8	0.1
Lackawanna	234,107	2.0	1	1.3	187	2.7
Lancaster	319,693	2.7	1	1.3	12	0.2
Lehigh	255,304	2.1	—	—	—	—
Luzerne	342,301	2.9	1	1.3	32	0.5
Northampton	214,368	1.8	1	1.3	144	2.1
Susquehanna	34,344	0.3	—	—	—	—
Washington	210,876	1.8	2	2.5	126	1.9
Wayne	29,581	0.2	—	—	—	—
Westmoreland	376,935	3.2	2	2.5	305	4.5
Wyoming	19,082	0.1	—	—	—	—
York	272,603	2.3	3	3.7	171	2.5
Category IV	3,136,992	26.8	23	29.1	1354	19.9
Armstrong	75,590	0.7	1	1.3	17	0.2
Beaver	208,418	1.8	2	2.5	216	3.2
Bedford	42,353	0.4	1	1.3	34	0.6
Blair	135,356	1.1	1	1.3	76	1.1
Bradford	57,962	0.5	—	—	—	—
Butler	127,941	1.1	2	2.5	76	1.1
Cambria	186,785	1.6	1	1.3	235	3.4

County Population			Programs		Alcoholics in Treatment	
County	1970 Pop.	%	No.	%	No.	%
Cameron	7,096	0.1	—	—	2	0.0
Carbon	50,573	0.5	1	1.3	5	0.1
Centre	99,267	0.8	—	—	—	—
Clarion	38,414	0.3	—	—	—	—
Clearfield	74,619	0.6	1	1.3	18	0.3
Clinton	37,721	0.3	—	—	—	—
Columbia	55,114	0.5	1	1.3	23	0.3
Crawford	81,342	0.7	1	1.3	135	2.0
Cumberland	158,177	1.3	2	2.5	41	0.7
Elk	37,770	0.3	—	—	7	0.1
Fayette	154,667	1.3	—	—	—	—
Forest	4,926	0.0	—	—	—	—
Franklin	100,833	1.0	—	—	—	—
Fulton	10,776	0.1	—	—	—	—
Huntingdon	39,108	0.3	—	—	—	—
Indiana	79,451	0.8	1	1.3	11	0.2
Jefferson	43,695	0.4	—	—	11	0.2
Juniata	16,712	0.1	—	—	—	—
Lawrence	107,374	1.0	—	—	—	—
Lebanon	99,665	0.8	—	—	—	—
Lycoming	113,296	1.0	—	—	—	—
McKean	51,915	0.4	1	1.3	42	0.6
Mercer	127,175	1.1	2	2.5	84	1.2
Mifflin	45,268	0.4	—	—	—	—
Monroe	45,422	0.4	1	1.3	22	0.3
Montour	16,508	0.1	1	1.3	37	0.5
Northumberland	99,190	0.8	—	—	—	—
Perry	28,615	0.2	—	—	9	0.1
Pike	11,818	0.1	—	—	5	0.1
Potter	16,395	0.1	—	—	7	0.1
Schuylkill	160,089	1.3	1	1.3	127	1.9
Synder	29,269	0.2	—	—	—	—
Somerset	76,037	0.7	—	—	66	1.0
Sullivan	5,691	0.1	—	—	—	—
Tioga	36,691	0.3	—	—	—	—
Union	28,603	0.2	1	1.3	10	0.1
Venango	62,353	0.5	1	1.3	17	0.2
Warren	47,682	0.5	1	1.3	21	0.3
Total	11,804,324	100.0	80	100.4	6805	100.2

TABLE A-2

Prevalence of Alcoholism and Prevalence of Treatment, By County

County	1970 pop.	Estimated Alcoholics[1]	Rate of Alcoholism per 10,000 pop.	Alcoholics in Treatment[2]	Rate in Treatment per 10,000 pop.	Rate of Estimated Alcoholics to Alcoholics in Treatment
Category I	3,553,625	445,357	1253	3127	9.0	142:1
Allegheny	1,605,016	211,162	1316	1831	11.4	115:1
Philadelphia	1,948,609	234,195	1202	1296	6.6	181:1
Category II	1,223,834	77,382	632	742	6.1	104:1
Delaware	600,035	45,002	750	443	7.3	102:1
Montgomery	623,799	32,380	519	299	4.7	108:1
Category III	3,889,873	235,086	604	1582	4.1	149:1
Adams	56,937	2,266	398	0	0	—
Berks	296,382	15,572	525	176	5.9	88:1
Bucks	415,471	11,530	277	46	1.1	251:1
Chester	278,311	8,697	312	222	8.0	39:1
Dauphin	233,834	14,448	645	46	1.9	314:1
Erie	263,654	17,898	679	107	4.0	167:1
Greene	35,090	4,259	1180	8	2.2	532:1
Lackawanna	234,107	34,199	1461	187	8.0	183:1
Lancaster	319,693	8,587	269	12	0.3	716:1

TABLE A-2

Prevalence of Alcoholism and Prevalence of Treatment, By County

County	1970 pop.	Estimated Alcoholics	Rate of Alcoholism per 10,000 pop.	Alcoholics in Treatment[2]	Rate in Treatment per 10,000 pop.	Rate of Estimated Alcoholics to Alcoholics in Treatment
Lehigh	255,304	13,914	545	0	0	—
Luzerne	342,301	39,946	1167	32	1.0	1248:1
Northampton	214,368	12,253	572	144	6.7	85:1
Susquehanna	34,344	792	231	0	0	—
Washington	210,876	15,867	752	126	6.0	126:1
Wayne	29,581	1,981	670	0	0	—
Westmoreland	376,935	23,502	624	305	8.0	77:1
Wyoming	19,082	518	271	0	0	—
York	272,603	8,857	325	171	6.3	52:1
Category IV	3,136,992	186,186	594	1354	4.3	137:1
Armstrong	75,590	6,664	882	17	2.2	392:1
Beaver	208,418	16,288	782	216	10.3	75:1
Bedford	42,353	1,973	466	66	15:6	30:1
Blair	135,356	8,850	654	76	5.6	116:1
Bradford	57,962	2,940	507	0	0	—
Butler	127,941	5,543	433	76	5.9	73:1
Cambria	186,785	9,513	509	235	12.5	40:1

TABLE A-2
Prevalence of Alcoholism and Prevalence of Treatment, By County

County	1970 pop.	Estimated Alcoholics[1]	Rate of Alcoholism per 10,000 pop.	Alcoholics in Treatment[2]	Rate in Treatment per 10,000 pop.	Rate of Estimated Alcoholics to Alcoholics in Treatment
Cameron	7,096	0	0	2	2.8	—
Carbon	50,573	4,203	831	5	1.0	841:1
Centre	99,267	1,779	179	0	0	—
Clarion	38,414	1,732	451	0	0	—
Clearfield	74,619	5,284	708	18	2.4	294:1
Clinton	37,721	2,103	558	0	0	—
Columbia	55,114	3,372	612	23	4.2	147:1
Crawford	81,342	6,502	799	135	16.5	48:1
Cumberland	158,177	5,747	363	41	2.6	140:1
Elk	37,770	4,563	1208	7	1.9	652:1
Fayette	154,667	17,448	1128	0	0	—
Forest	4,926	213	432	0	0	—
Franklin	100,833	1,031	102	0	0	—
Fulton	10,776	48	45	0	0	—
Huntingdon	39,108	1,010	258	0	0	—
Indiana	79,451	1,633	206	11	1.4	148:1
Jefferson	43.695	881	202	11	2.5	80:1

TABLE A-2

Prevalence of Alcoholism and Prevalence of Treatment, By County

County	1970 pop.	Estimated Alcoholics[1]	Rate of Alcoholism per 10,000 pop.	Alcoholics in Treatment[2]	Rate in Treatment per 10,000 pop.	Rate of Estimated Alcoholics to Alcoholics in Treatment
Juniata	16,712	233	139	0	0	—
Lawrence	107,374	7,879	734	0	0	—
Mercer	127,175	9,080	714	85	6.6	107:1
Mifflin	45,268	485	107	0	0	—
Monroe	45,422	2,590	570	22	4.8	118:1
Montour	16,508	239	145	37	22.4	6:1
Northumberland	99,190	6,703	676	0	0	—
Perry	28,615	601	210	9	3.1	67:1
Pike	11,818	1,074	909	5	4.2	215:1
Potter	16,395	0	0	7	5.3	—
Schuylkill	160,089	21,966	1366	127	7.9	172:1
Snyder	29,269	0	0	0	0	—
Somerset	76,037	5,599	736	34	4.5	165:1
Sullivan	5,961	887	1488	0	0	—

TABLE A-2

Prevalence of Alcoholism and Prevalence of Treatment, By County

County	1970 pop.	Estimated Alcoholics[1]	Rate of Alcoholism per 10,000 pop.	Alcoholics in Treatment[2]	Rate in Treatment per 10,000 pop.	Rate of Estimated Alcoholics to Alcoholics in Treatment
Tioga	59,691	1,696	427	0	0	—
Union	28,603	0	0	10	3.5	—
Venango	62,353	2,817	452	17	2.7	166:1
Warren	47,682	1,472	309	21	4.4	70:1
Total	11,804,324	944,011	800	6,805	5.7	139:1

[1] These figures are based on the Brenner formula, a transformation of cirrhosis deaths. The prevalence of alcoholism in Pennsylvania (1970) as estimated by the Brenner formula is 50% higher than that estimated by the Schaps-Rubin survey, but for the present purposes this does not appear to be a serious threat to the validity of the conclusions.

[2] Since four-fifths of all alcoholics in treatment receive treatment in their county of residence, the numbers of alcoholics in treatment per county was calculated by adding the patient census of the programs located in each county. This will result in some error, since a few patients cross county lines to receive treatment.

Table A-3

Number of Male Alcoholics in Treatment by County and Race

County	County Population — Male				Males in Treatment			
	White	Non-White	Total	% Non-White	White	Non-White	Total	% Non-White
Category I	1,299,507	381,154	1,680,661	22.6	1270	1260	2530	49.8
Allegheny	692,255	70,233	762,488	9.2	907	457	1364	33.5
Philadelphia	607,252	310,921	918,173	33.8	363	803	1166	68.9
Category II	555,019	33,695	588,714	5.7	434	138	572	24.1
Delaware	267,055	21,348	288,403	7.4	259	79	338	23.4
Montgomery	287,964	12,347	300,311	4.1	175	59	234	25.2
Category III	1,819,515	56,066	1,875,581	3.0	1107	188	1295	14.5
Adams	27,704	374	28,078	1.3	—	—	—	—
Berks	138,717	3,497	142,214	2.4	117	26	143	18.2
Bucks	200,677	4,662	205,339	2.2	26	3	29	10.3
Chester	125,967	11,059	137,026	8.0	134	52	186	38.8
Dauphin	93,506	12,682	106,188	11.9	27	11	38	28.9
Erie	122,533	4,508	127,041	3.5	49	45	94	47.9
Greene	17,223	154	17,377	0.8	8	0	8	0.0
Lackawanna	109,132	633	109,765	0.5	160	8	168	4.8
Lancaster	151,917	2,892	154,809	1.8	12	0	12	0.0
Lehigh	121,269	1,448	122,717	1.1	—	—	—	—
Luzerne	159,963	1,077	161,040	0.6	21	0	21	0.0

Table A-3

Number of Male Alcoholics in Treatment
by County and Race

County	County Population — Male				Males in Treatment			
	White	Non-White	Total	% Non-White	White	Non-White	Total	% Non-White
Northampton	103,200	1,938	105,138	1.8	115	2	117	1.7
Susquehanna	16,970	33	17,003	0.1	—	—	—	—
Washington	98,562	3,808	102,370	3.7	98	1	99	1
Wayne	14,486	318	14,804	2.1	—	—	—	—
Westmoreland	179,522	3,188	182,710	1.7	238	10	248	4.0
Wyoming	9,415	25	9,440	0.2	—	—	—	—
York	128,752	3,770	132,522	2.8	102	30	132	22.7
Category IV	1,495,455	25,003	1,520,458	1.6	1039	69	1108	6.2
Armstrong	36,198	422	32,620	1.1	12	0	12	0.0
Beaver	95,697	5,733	101,430	5.6	165	20	185	10.8
Bedford	20,597	70	20,667	0.3	29	0	29	0.0
Blair	63,361	550	63,911	0.8	62	1	63	1.6
Bradford	28,139	98	28,237	0.3	—	—	—	—
Butler	61,992	322	62,314	0.5	62	0	62	0.0
Cambria	88,119	1,809	89,928	2.0	153	11	164	6.7
Cameron	3,346	13	3,359	0.3	2	1	2	0.0
Carbon	24,207	77	24,284	0.3	4	0	4	0.0
Centre	50,870	1,190	52,060	2.2	—	—	—	—

Clarion	18,647	48	18,695	0.2	—	—	—	—
Clearfield	36,067	115	36,182	0.3	15	0	15	0.0
Clinton	18,295	48	18,343	0.2	—	—	—	—
Columbia	26,401	74	26,475	0.2	20	0	20	0.0
Crawford	39,133	556	39,689	1.4	116	6	122	4.9
Cumberland	75,459	1,304	76,763	1.6	27	4	31	12.9
Elk	18,362	18	18,380	0.1	5	0	5	0.0
Fayette	71,169	3,297	74,466	4.4	—	—	—	—
Forest	2,440	21	2,461	0.8	—	—	—	—
Franklin	47,487	956	48,443	1.9	—	—	—	—
Fulton	5,332	31	5,363	0.5	—	—	—	—
Huntingdon	18,693	672	19,365	3.4	—	—	—	—
Indiana	37,872	281	38,153	0.7	11	0	11	0.0
Jefferson	20,867	23	20,890	0.1	10	0	10	0.0
Juniata	8,166	3	8,169	0.1	—	—	—	—
Lawrence	50,523	1,425	51,948	2.7	—	—	—	—
Lebanon	48,366	280	48,646	0.5	—	—	—	—
Lycoming	53,641	706	54,347	1.2	—	—	—	—
McKean	24,746	80	24,826	0.3	29	0	29	0.0
Mercer	59,599	2,622	62,221	4.2	65	8	73	11.0
Mifflin	21,438	63	21,501	0.2	—	—	—	—
Monroe	21,385	376	21,752	1.6	17	0	17	0.0
Montour	7,506	55	7,561	0.7	24	6	30	20.0
Northumberland	46,798	79	46,868	0.1	—	—	—	—
Perry	14,149	45	14,194	0.3	7	0	7	0.0
Pike	5,711	20	5,731	0.3	4	0	4	0.0
Potter	8,005	40	8,045	0.4	5	0	5	0.0
Schuylkill	75,980	215	76,195	0.2	103	10	113	8.8

Table A-3

Number of Male Alcoholics in Treatment
by County and Race

County	County Population — Male				Males in Treatment			
	White	Non-White	Total	% Non-White	White	Non-White	Total	% Non-White
Snyder	14,357	101	14,458	0.7	—	—	—	—
Somerset	36,967	91	37,058	0.2	61	0	61	0.0
Sullivan	2,964	12	2,976	0.4	—	—	—	—
Tioga	19,181	68	19,249	0.3	—	—	—	—
Union	14,214	709	14,923	4.7	7	1	8	12.5
Venango	29,899	223	30,122	0.7	13	0	13	0.0
Warren	23,119	71	23,190	0.3	11	2	13	15.4
Total	5,169,496	495,918	5,665,414	8.7	3,850	1,655	5,505	30.1

Table A-4

Place of Residence of Alcoholics in Treatment, By County in Which Treatment Is Received

County	No. Alcoholics treated in this county	% from Penna.	% from this county	% from Phila.	% from Allegheny Co.
Category I	3127	91.9	88.1	—	—
Allegheny	1831	86.3	80.1	0.1	80.1
Philadelphia	1296	99.8	99.3	99.3	2.0
Category II	742	93.8	75.1	8.9	0.0
Delaware	443	92.3	89.4	1.6	0.0
Montgomery	299	95.3	53.8	19.7	0.0
Category III	1582	94.2	67.8	5.4	1.5
Adams	—	—	—	—	—
Berks	176	92.0	64.2	5.1	5.1
Bucks	46	69.6	15.2	28.3	2.2
Chester	222	88.7	68.9	21.2	0.0
Dauphin	46	100.0	67.4	0.0	2.2
Erie	107	91.6	82.2	0.0	0.0
Greene	—	—	—	—	—
Lackawanna	187	100.0	100.0	0.0	0.0
Lancaster	12	100.0	8.3	50.0	8.3
Lehigh	—	—	—	—	—
Luzerne	32	100.0	100.0	0.0	0.0
Northampton	144	79.2	41.7	0.0	0.0
Susquehanna	—	—	—	—	—
Washington	134	100.0	31.3	7.5	7.5
Wayne	—	—	—	—	—
Westmoreland	305	100.0	62.3	0.0	0.0
Wyoming	—	—	—	—	—

Table A-4

Place of Residence of Alcoholics in Treatment, By County in Which Treatment Is Received

County	No. Alcoholics treated in this county	% from Penna.	% from this county	% from Phila.	% from Allegheny Co.
York	171	100.0	98.2	0.0	0.0
Category IV	1354	99.3	79.1	0.8	3.1
Armstrong	17	100.0	100.0	0.0	0.0
Beaver	216	96.8	68.1	0.0	18.5
Bedford	—	—	—	—	—
Blair	76	100.0	89.5	0.0	0.0
Bradford	—	—	—	—	—
Butler	76	100.0	92.1	0.0	0.0
Cambria	235	98.7	85.9	0.0	0.0
Cameron	—	—	—	—	—
Carbon	—	—	—	—	—
Centre	—	—	—	—	—
Clarion	—	—	—	—	—
Clinton	—	—	—	—	—
Clearfield	29	100.0	62.1	0.0	0.0
Columbia	23	100.0	91.3	0.0	0.0
Crawford	135	100.0	100.0	0.0	0.0
Cumberland	50	100.0	76.0	6.0	0.0
Elk	—	—	—	—	—
Fayette	—	—	—	—	—
Forest	—	—	—	—	—
Franklin	—	—	—	—	—
Fulton	—	—	—	—	—
Huntingdon	—	—	—	—	—

Table A-4

Place of Residence of Alcoholics in Treatment, By County in Which Treatment Is Received

County	No. Alcoholics treated in this county	% from Penna.	% from this county	% from Phila.	% from Allegheny Co.
Jefferson	—	—	—	—	—
Juniata	—	—	—	—	—
Lawrence	—	—	—	—	—
Lebanon	—	—	—	—	—
Lycoming	—	—	—	—	—
McKean	58	100.0	63.8	1.7	0.0
Mercer	84	100.0	97.6	0.0	0.0
Mifflin	—	—	—	—	—
Monroe	32	100.0	68.8	0.0	0.0
Montour	37	100.0	0.0	16.2	0.0
Northumberland	—	—	—	—	—
Perry	—	—	—	—	—
Pike	—	—	—	—	—
Potter	—	—	—	—	—
Schuylkill	127	100.0	100.0	0.0	0.0
Snyder	—	—	—	—	—
Somerset	100	100.0	66.0	0.0	0.0
Sullivan	—	—	—	—	—
Tioga	—	—	—	—	—
Union	10	100.0	0.0	10.0	0.0
Venango	17	100.0	100.0	0.0	0.0
Warren	21	100.0	9.5	0.0	0.0
Total	6805	6446	5458	1451	1597
		94.7%	80.2%	21.3%	23.5%

Table A-5

Number of Staff and Staff/Patient Ratio of Treatment Components

Components	Full-time		Part-time+		F-T Professionals Other than Physicians		F-T Recovered Alcoholics		Full-time Physicians		Part-time Physicians		Full-time Non-treatment †		Patients
	No.	Ratio	No.	Ratio	No.	Ratio	No.	Ratio	No.	Ratio	No.	Ratio	No.	Ratio	
I	21	1:2	10	1:3	8	1:4	2	1:16	2	1:16	2	1:16	4	1:8	32
II	0	—	0	—	0	—	0	—	0	—	0	—	0	—	0
III	143	1:3	54	1:7	49	1:8	56	1:7	4	1:92	6	1:61	38	1:10	368
IV	33	1:7	3	1:74	9	1:25	14	1:16	0	—	2	1:111	5	1:44	221
V	112	1:27	113	1:26	61	1:49	12	1:248	2	1:1488	43	1:69	33	1:90	2976
VI	0	—	5	1:4	0	—	0	—	0	—	0	—	0	—	21
I, III	2	1:7	5	1:3	0	—	2	1:7	0	—	2	1:7	0	—	14
I, V	65	1:22	15	1:96	36	1:40	8	1:180	1	1:1440	8	1:180	9	1:160	1440
III, IV	112*	1:1	50	1:2	35	1:3	25	1:5	4	1:29	11	1:11	49	1:2	116
III, V	7	1:14	1	1:100	3	1:33	3	1:33	0	—	0	—	1	1:100	100
III, VI	23	1:2	19	1:2	1	1:37	1	1:37	1	1:37	4	1:9	1	1:37	37
IV, V	14	1:4	20	1:3	14	1:4	4	1:15	0	—	6	1:10	2	1:29	58
IV, VI	7	1:19	2	1:32	3	1:21	4	1:16	0	—	1	1:63	0	—	63
I, III, V	64	1:4	36	1:8	10	1:28	5	1:55	5	1:55	7	1:40	18	1:15	277
I, V, VI	14	1:4	3	1:18	5	1:11	2	1:27	0	—	1	1:53	1	1:53	53
I, II, III, V	21	1:16	4	1:82	14	1:23	2	1:163	1	1:326	2	1:163	2	1:163	326
II, III, IV, V	6*	1:12	7	1:10	4	1:18	1	1:71	0	—	3	1:24	1	1:71	71
I, II, III, IV, V	96	1:7	18	1:35	36	1:18	61	1:10	2	1:316	15	1:37	9	1:70	632
TOTAL	740	1:9	365	1:19	288	1:24	202	1:34	22	1:309	113	1:60	173	1:39	6805

\+ This category includes all part-time employees—i.e. professionals, recovered alcoholics, and non-treatment staff.

† This category includes all full-time staff not directly involved in treatment, i.e. secretarial, custodial, etc.

* In two programs drug addicts and alcoholics were treated together. Therefore, by definition, full-time staff members divided their time equally between these two groups of patients. For that reason, the number of full-time staff in these two programs was divided in half.

Appendix B

PROGRAM DIRECTORY

AL-ASSIST*

Address:	907 Pine Street Philadelphia, Pa. 19107
Director:	Quinton Brown
Phone:	(215) 829-3417

Agency Profile

Governing auspices:	Private corporation
Source of funds:	Federal
Type of agency:	Out-patient
Treatment elements:	V
Type of facility:	Store front
Waiting list:	None
Treatment objectives:	Life without alcohol
Type of alcoholic:	Chronic non-skid row
Referrals from:	Walk-in
AA:	No

Admission Information

1. Geographical area — Philadelphia
2. Emergency service — Refer to neighborhood health centre
3. Type of alcohol abused — Wine
4. Age — No exclusions
5. Sex — No exclusions
6. Payment for service — None required
7. Other — None

* This is a sample entry from the program directory. The complete directory is available from the Addiction Research Foundation of Ontario, 33 Russell Street, Toronto, Ontario, M5S 2S1.

Appendix C

RELEVANT LEGISLATION

1. Proposed Public Inebriate Act
2. "Hughes Act" (P.L.91-616 as amended)

The General Assembly of Pennsylvania

HOUSE BILL No. 135 — Session of 1975

Introduced by Mr. DiCarlo, Mrs. Crawford, Mrs. Kelly, Messrs. M.E. Miller, Jr., Rhodes, Lincoln, McCall, Zwikl, Berlin, Milliron, Laughlin, Hill, Mrs. Toll, Messrs. Reed, Oliver, Tayoun, Myers, Green, Mrs. Fawcett, Messrs. Hammock, Fisher, Haskell, Wagner, Taddonio, Gallagher, R.W. Wilt and Cole, January 28, 1975.

As reported from Committee on Health and Welfare, House of Representatives, as amended, May 27, 1975

AN ACT

Amending the act of April 14, 1972 (P.L.221, No.63), entitled "An act establishing the Governor's Council On Drug and Alcohol Abuse; imposing duties on the council to develop and coordinate the implementation of a comprehensive health, education and rehabilitation program for the prevention and treatment of drug and alcohol abuse and drug and alcohol dependence; providing for emergency medical treatment; providing for treatment and rehabilitation alternatives to the criminal process for drug and alcohol dependence; and making repeals," further providing for the establishment of a special alcohol treatment system, providing powers and duties to designate and regulate facilities and designated persons, providing authority for grants and contracts and making repeals.

The General Assembly of the Commonwealth of Pennsylvania hereby enacts as follows:

Section 1. Subsection (b) of section 2, act of April 14, 1972 (P.L.221, No.63), known as the "Pennsylvania Drug and Alcohol Abuse Control Act," is amended by adding definitions to read:

Section 2. Definitions:

(b) As used in this act:

"Administrator" means the person in charge of the operation of a facility, or his designee.

"Alcoholic" means a person suffering from alcoholism.

"Alcoholism" means a medically diagnosed disease characterized by chronic habitual or periodic consumption of alcoholic beverages resulting in the (i) substantial interference with an individual's social or economic functions in the community, or (ii) the loss of powers of self-control with respect to the use of such beverages.

***

"Designated person" means a person designated by the council for specific purposes under section 10 of this act. Police officers may be designated persons.

"Facility" means a facility designated by the council to provide emergency medical services, and/or detoxification and other necessary care to persons under section 10 of this act. Criteria for facilities shall be established by regulation and published pursuant to the Commonwealth Documents Law.

***

"Incapacitated" means that a person, as a result of the use of alcohol, is unconscious or has his judgment otherwise so impaired that he is incapable of realizing and making a rational decision with respect to his need for treatment.

***

"PROJECT" MEANS THE ADMINISTRATIVE STRUCTURE WHICH HAS AS ITS GOAL THE DELIVERY OF DRUG OR ALCOHOL SERVICES. A PROJECT MAY HAVE ONE OR MORE FACILITIES.

Section 2. SUBSECTION (A) OF SECTION 4 Of the act is amended by adding CLAUSES to read: Section 4. COUNCIL'S POWERS AND RESPONSIBILITIES. — (A) THE COUNCIL SHALL DEVELOP AND ADOPT A STATE PLAN FOR THE CONTROL, PREVENTION, TREATMENT, REHABILITATION, RESEARCH, EDUCATION, AND TRAINING ASPECTS OF DRUG AND ALCOHOL ABUSE AND DEPENDENCE PROBLEMS. THE STATE PLAN SHALL INCLUDE, BUT NOT BE LIMITED TO, PROVISION FOR:

(21) *The council shall have the power to issue grants to, and to contract with public and private agencies.*

(22) *Financial obligations for services as described in Section 10 of this act shall be in accordance with Section 13 of this act.*

(23) *The council shall promulgate such rules and regulations pursuant to law as may be necessary to carry into effect the provisions of this act.*

Section 3. Section 10 of the act is amended to read:

Section 10. General.—(a) Drug and alcohol abuse or dependence shall be regarded as a health problem, sickness, physical and mental illness, disease, disability, or similar term, for purposes of all legislation relating to health, welfare, and rehabilitation programs, services, funds and other benefits.

(b) *Any person who voluntarily applies for treatment at a facility or is brought to a facility in accordance with this section shall be afforded treatment there or at another facility* OR PROJECT.

(1) *Prior to the admission of any person into a facility and within a reasonable time from arrival at said facility, the administrator shall cause the person to be evaluated by* A PERSON QUALIFIED AS A RESULT OF TRAINING OR EXPERIENCE *in alcoholism diagnosis. If there is any concern about the health or the immediate needs of such person, he shall be immediately examined by a physician. If upon said evaluation or examination, a determination is made that the person is incapacitated and adequate and appropriate treatment is available, he shall be admitted. If any person is not admitted for the reason that adequate and appropriate treatment is not available at the facility, the administrator shall make all necessary arrangements with a facility at which adequate and appropriate treatment is available and then shall refer the person thereto. In the event that a person is not admitted to a facility, and has no available funds, the administrator shall arrange for the person to be assisted to his residence, or the residence of a friend or family. In the event that no residence is available, the person shall be assisted to a place where proper shelter shall be provided him.*

(2) *Any person admitted to a facility shall neither be detained nor receive treatment at the facility without his voluntary and informed consent: provided, in the opinion of the* PERSON QUALIFIED AS A RESULT OF TRAINING OR EXPERIENCE IN ALCOHOLISM DIAGNOSIS AND EMPLOYED BY THE FACILITY, *the person has the requisite capacity to give such consent. All persons shall be given adequate notice of their right to leave the facility and any person who wants to leave may do so. If the person does not have the requisite capacity to so consent, the person shall not be detained for a period greater than 72 hours after being admitted unless he is committed under the provisions of the act of October 20, 1966 (3rd Sp.Sess., P.L.96, No.61,) known as the "Mental Health and Mental Retardation Act of 1966." Patients may* VOLUNTARILY *consent to remain in treatment for* LONGER THAN 72 HOURS IF THE PERSON QUALIFIED AS A RESULT OF TRAINING OR EXPERIENCE IN ALCOHOLISM DIAGNOSIS DEEMS IT APPROPRIATE.

(3) *When a person is admitted to a facility, his family shall be notified as soon thereafter as possible, but the facility is not required to do so if the person requests otherwise. Any person who is transported to a facility or from one facility to another or from a facility to his residence shall be transported in accordance with the regulations promulgated by the council regarding such transportation.*

(4) *Upon discharge from or upon leaving a facility, the patient shall be encouraged to seek appropriate aftercare treatment.*

(c) *Incapacitated persons.*

(1) *Any person who, in a public place, is incapacitated may be assisted by a designated person with or without his consent, forthwith to a facility. If no facility is readily available and the person appears to be in need of emergency*

medical services and/or is unconscious, he shall be taken to an emergency medical facility. The designated person shall make every reasonable effort to protect the health and safety of the person.

(2) *To determine, for purposes of this subsection only, whether or not such person is incapacitated, the designated person may request the person to submit to any reasonable test including, but not limited to, tests of his coordination, coherence of speech and breath. No such records, results or information may be used to initiate or substantiate criminal charges against a patient under any circumstances.*

(3) *Any person assisted by a designated person to a facility shall receive treatment in accordance with subsection* (b).

(4) *A person assisted to a facility by a designated person and/or the police pursuant to the provisions of this subsection, shall not be considered to have been arrested, or to have been charged with any crime; however, an entry of assistance shall be made indicating the date, time and place of assistance, which record shall not be treated for any purposes as an arrest or criminal record. The police or a designated person who is acting in compliance with this subsection shall be considered acting in the course of their official duty, and shall not incur any increase in criminal or civil liability for their actions pursuant to this subsection.*

(d) *Criminal law limitations.*

(1) *No county, municipality, or other political subdivision may adopt or enforce a local law, ordinance, resolution, or rule having the force of law that includes being a common drunkard, or being found in an intoxicated condition as one of the elements of the offense giving rise to a criminal or civil penalty or sanction.*

(2) *No county, municipality, or other political subdivision may interpret or apply any law, ordinance, resolution or rule having the force of law to circumvent the provision of clause (1) of this subsection.*

(3) *Nothing in this act affects any law, ordinance, resolution, or rule against drunken driving, driving under the influence of alcohol, or other similar offense involving the operation of a vehicle, aircraft, boat, machinery or concerning the sale, purchase, dispensing, possession and use of alcoholic beverages at stated times and places or by a particular class of persons.*

(e) *THE COUNCIL SHALL ESTABLISH RULES AND REGULATIONS SETTING THE STANDARDS FOR THE DESIGNATION OF FACILITIES TO BE USED FOR DETOXIFICATION OF PERSONS; FOR QUALIFICATIONS OF PERSONS AS "DESIGNATED PERSONS"; AND FOR THE QUALIFICATIONS AND TRAINING NECESSARY FOR A PERSON TO BE DEEMED A "PERSON QUALIFIED AS A RESULT OF TRAINING OR EXPERIENCE IN ALCOHOLISM DIAGNOSIS." SUCH RULES AND REGULATIONS SHALL BE ADOPTED AND PUBLISHED IN ACCORDANCE WITH THE COMMONWEALTH DOCUMENTS LAW. Facilities offering emergency medical services shall meet standards established by the Department of Health.*

Section 4. (a) There shall be established a Joint Committee of the Public Health and Welfare Committees of the Senate and the House of Representatives including representatives of the council. The committee shall be composed of nine persons and selected in the following manner:

(1) The President *pro tempore* of the Senate shall select three members: two from the majority and one from the minority.

(2) The Speaker of the House of Representatives shall select three members: two from the majority and one from the minority.

(3) The chairman of the council shall serve and shall select two additional members of the council.

(b) The said committee is constituted solely for the purpose of determining the appropriate date or dates and phases for the implementation of this act. When the said sole purpose of the committee has been fulfilled, the committee shall be dissolved. SINCE THE DETERMINATION OF IMPLEMENTATION DATES IS CONTINGENT UPON A PLAN OF IMPLEMENTATION, THE COMMITTEE SHALL NOT FINALLY DETERMINE THE DATES OF IMPLEMENTATION FOR THIS ACT UNTIL IT HAS HAD THE BENEFIT OF THE IMPLEMENTATION PLAN TO BE SUBMITTED BY THE COUNCIL AS MANDATED IN SECTION 4 OF THIS AMENDATORY ACT.

SECTION 5. THE COUNCIL SHALL SUBMIT TO THE PRESIDENT PRO TEM OF THE SENATE AND THE SPEAKER OF THE HOUSE, FOR REVIEW AND ANALYSIS BY THE SUBSTANTIVE COMMITTEES OF EACH HOUSE AND THE JOINT COMMITTEE ON THE PUBLIC HEALTH AND WELFARE AS CREATED IN SECTION 3, A DETAILED PLAN FOR THE IMPLEMENTATION OF THE PROVISIONS OF THIS ACT. THE PLAN SHALL INCLUDE A DETAILED ANALYTICAL ESTIMATE OF ALL DIRECT AND INDIRECT IMPLEMENTING AND OPERATING COSTS AND THE AVAILABILITY OF FEDERAL MATCHING MONEYS AND OTHER POSSIBLE SOURCES OF REVENUE TO EFFECT THE INTENT OF THIS ACT. THE COST ESTIMATES SHALL BE PROJECTED THROUGH FIVE CONSECUTIVE FISCAL YEARS COMMENCING WITH THE FISCAL YEAR BEGINNING JULY 1, 1976. THE PLAN OF IMPLEMENTATION SHALL BE SUBMITTED TO THE PRESIDENT PRO TEMPORE AND SPEAKER NO LATER THAN ONE YEAR FROM THE EFFECTIVE DATE OF THIS ACT.

Section 6. (a) The following acts and parts of acts are repealed to the extent indicated:

(1) Section 29, act of March 31, 1856 (P.L.200, No.233), entitled "An act to Regulate the Sale of Intoxicating Liquors," absolutely.

(2) Section 591, act of May 1, 1933 (P.L.103, No.69), reenacted and amended July 10, 1947 (PL.1481, No.567), known as "The Second

Class Township Code," in so far as it relates to drunkenness.

(3) Section 1121, act of February 1, 1966 (1965 P.L.1656, No.581), known as "The Borough Code," in so far as it relates to drunkenness.

(4) Section 5505 of Title 18 of the Pennsylvania Consolidated Statutes (relating to public drunkenness), added December 6, 1972 (P.L.1482, No.334), absolutely.

(b) All other acts and parts of acts are hereby repealed in so far as inconsistent with provisions of this act.

Section 7. This act shall take effect in 60 days EXCEPT SECTION 6 OF THIS ACT WHICH SHALL TAKE EFFECT UPON THE DATE FOR IMPLEMENTING THIS ACT FIXED BY THE COMMITTEE CREATED IN SECTION 3.

93rd Congress
2nd Session

COMPREHENSIVE ALCOHOL ABUSE AND ALCOHOLISM PREVENTION, TREATMENT, AND REHABILITATION ACT OF 1970,
AS AMENDED

Including Changes Made by Public Law 93-282,
May 14, 1974

Prepared for the
SUBCOMMITTEE ON ALCOHOLISM AND NARCOTICS
of the
COMMITTEE ON LABOR AND PUBLIC WELFARE
UNITED STATES SENATE

December 1974

SHORT TITLE

Section 1. This Act may be cited as the "Comprehensive Alcohol Abuse and Alcoholism Prevention, Treatment, and Rehabilitation Act of 1970".

FINDINGS AND PURPOSE

Sec. 2 (a) The Congress finds that—

(1) alcohol is one of the most dangerous drugs and the drug most frequently abused in the United States;

(2) of the Nation's estimated ninety-five million drinkers, at least nine million, or 7 per centum of the adult population, are alcohol abusers and alcoholics;

(3) problem drinking costs the national economy at least $15,000,-000,000 annually in lost working time, medical and public assistance expenditures, and police and court costs;

(4) alcohol abuse is found with increasing frequency among persons who are multiple-drug abusers and among former heroin users who are being treated in methadone maintenance programs;

(5) alcohol abuse is being discovered among growing numbers of youth; and

(6) alcoholism is an illness requiring treatment and rehabilitation through the assistance of a broad range of community health and social services, and with the cooperation of law enforcement agencies.

(b) It is the policy of the United States and the purpose of this Act to (1) approach alcohol abuse and alcoholism from a comprehensive community care standpoint, and (2) meet the problems of alcohol abuse and alcoholism not only through Federal assistance to the States but also through direct Federal assistance to community-based programs meeting the urgent needs of special populations and developing methods for diverting problem drinkers from criminal justice systems into prevention and treatment programs.

TITLE I—NATIONAL INSTITUTE ON ALCOHOL ABUSE AND ALCOHOLISM

Establishment of the Institute

Sec. 101. (a) There is established the National Institute on Alcohol Abuse and Alcoholism (hereafter in this Act referred to as the "Institute") to administer the programs and authorities assigned to the Secretary of Health, Education, and Welfare (hereafter in this Act referred to as the "Secretary") by this Act and part C of the Community Mental Health Centers Act. The Secretary, acting through the Institute, shall, in carrying out the purposes of sections 301 and 303 of the Public Health Service Act with respect to alcohol abuse and alcoholism, develop and conduct comprehensive health, education, training, research, and planning programs for the prevention and treatment of alcohol abuse and alcoholism and for the rehabilitation of alcohol abusers and alcoholics. The Secretary shall carry out through the Institute the administrative and financial management, policy development and planning, evaluation, and public information functions which are required for the implementation of such programs and authorities.

(b) (1) The Institute shall be under the direction of a Director who shall be appointed by the Secretary.

(2) The Director, with the approval of the Secretary, may employ and prescribe the functions of such officers and employees, including attorneys, as are necessary to administer the programs to be carried out through the Institute.

(c) The programs to be carried out through the Institute shall be administered so as to encourage the broadest possible participation of professionals and paraprofessionals in the fields of medicine, science, the social sciences, and other related disciplines.

Reports by the Secretary

Sec. 102, The Secretary shall—

(1) submit an annual report to Congress which shall include a description of the actions taken, services provided, and funds expended under this Act and part C of the Community Mental Health Centers Act, an evaluation of the effectiveness of such actions, services, and expenditures of funds, and such other information as the Secretary considers appropriate;

(2) submit to Congress on or before the expiration of the one-year period beginning on the date of enactment of this Act and every three years thereafter a report (A) containing current information on the health consequences of using alcoholic beverages, and (B) containing such recommendations for legislation and administrative action as he may deem appropriate;

(3) submit such additional reports as may be requested by the President of the United States or by Congress;

(4) submit to the President of the United States and to Congress such recommendations as will further the prevention, treatment, and control of alcohol abuse and alcoholism; and

(5) submit to Congress on or before the end of each calendar year a report on the extent to which other Federal programs and departments are concerned and dealing effectively with the problems of alcohol abuse and alcoholism.

Before submitting a report under paragraph (5), the Secretary shall give each department and agency of the Government which (or a program of which) is referred to in the report he proposes to submit under such paragraph an opportunity to comment on the proposed report; and the Secretary shall include in the report submitted to Congress under such paragraph the comments received by him from any such department or agency within 30 days from the date the proposed report was submitted to such department or agency.

Interagency Committee on Federal Activities for Alcohol Abuse and Alcoholism

Sec. 103. (a) The Secretary shall establish an Interagency Committee on Federal Activities for Alcohol Abuse and Alcoholism (hereinafter in this section referred to as the "Committee"). The Committee shall (1) evaluate the adequacy and technical soundness of all Federal programs and activities which relate to alcoholism and alcohol abuse and provide for the communication and exchange of information necessary to maintain the coordination and effectiveness of such programs and activities, and (2) seek to coordinate efforts undertaken to deal with alcohol abuse and alcoholism in carrying out Federal health, welfare, rehabilitation, highway safety, law enforcement, and economic opportunity laws.

(b) The Secretary or the Director of the National Institute on Alcohol Abuse and Alcoholism (or the Director's designee) shall serve as Chairman of the Committee, the membership of which shall include (1) appropriate scientific, medical, or technical representation from the Department of Transportation, the Department of Justice, the Department of Defense, the Veterans' Administration, and such other Federal agencies and offices (including appropriate agencies and offices of the Department of Health, Education, and Welfare) as the Secretary determines administer programs directly affecting alcoholism and alcohol abuse, and (2) five individuals from the general public appointed by the Secretary from individuals who by virtue of their training or experience are particularly qualified to participate in the performance of the Committee's functions. The Committee shall meet at the call of the Chairman, but not less often than four times a year.

(c) Each appointed member of the Committee shall be appointed for a term of four years, except that—

(1) any member appointed to fill a vacancy occurring prior to the expiration of the term for which his predecessor was appointed shall be appointed for the remainder of such term; and

(2) of the members first appointed, two shall be appointed for a term of four years, two shall be appointed for a term of three years, and one shall be appointed for a term of one year, as designated by the Secretary at the time of appointment.

Appointed members may serve after the expiration of their terms until their successors have taken office.

(d) Appointed members of the Committee shall receive for each day they are engaged in the performance of the functions of the Committee compensation at rates not to exceed the daily equivalent of the annual rate in effect for grade GS-18 of the General Schedule, including traveltime; and all members, while so serving away from their homes or regular places of business, may be allowed travel expenses, including per diem in lieu of subsistence, in the same manner as such expenses are authorized by section 5703 of title 5, United States Code, for persons in the Government service employed intermittently.

(e) The secretary shall make available to the Committee such staff, information, and other assistance as it may require to carry out its activities effectively.

TITLE II—ALCOHOL ABUSE AND ALCOHOLISM PREVENTION, TREATMENT, AND REHABILITATION PROGRAMS FOR FEDERAL CIVILIAN EMPLOYEES

Alcohol Abuse and Alcoholism Among Federal Civilian Employees

Sec. 201. (a) The Civil Service Commission shall be responsible for developing and maintaining, in cooperation with the Secretary and with other Federal agencies and departments, appropriate prevention, treatment, and rehabilitation programs and services for alcohol abuse and alcoholism among Federal civilian employees, consistent with the purposes of this Act. Such policies and services shall make optimal use of existing governmental facilities, services, and skills.

(b) The Secretary, acting through the Institute, shall be responsible for fostering similar alcohol abuse and alcoholism prevention, treatment, and rehabilitation programs and services in State and local governments and in private industry.

(c) (1) No person may be denied or deprived of Federal civilian employment or a Federal professional or other license or right solely on the ground of prior alcohol abuse or prior alcoholism.

(2) This subsection shall not apply to employment (A) in the Central Intelligence Agency, the Federal Bureau of Investigation, the National Security Agency, or any other department or agency of the Federal Government designated for purposes of national security by the President, or (B) in any position in any department or agency of the Federal Government, not referred to in clause (A), which position is determined pursuant to regulations prescribed by the head of such agency or department to be a sensitive position.

(d) This title shall not be construed to prohibit the dismissal from employment of a Federal civilian employee who cannot properly function in his employment.

TITLE III—FEDERAL ASSISTANCE FOR STATE AND LOCAL PROGRAMS

Part A—Grants to States

Authorization for Formula Grants

Sec. 301. There are authorized to be appropriated $40,000,000 for the fiscal year ending June 30, 1971, $60,000,000 for the fiscal year ending June 30, 1972, $80,000,000 for each of the next two fiscal years, $80,000,000 for the fiscal year ending June 30, 1975, and $80,000,000 for the fiscal year ending June 30, 1976, for grants to States to assist them in planning, establishing, maintaining, coordinating, and evaluating projects for the development of more effective prevention, treatment, and rehabilitation programs to deal with alcohol abuse and alcoholism. For purposes of this part, the term "State" includes the District of Columbia, the Virgin Islands, the Commonwealth of Puerto Rico, Guam, American Samoa, and the Trust Territory of the Pacific Islands, in addition to the fifty States.

State Allotment

Sec. 302. (a) For each fiscal year the Secretary shall, in accordance with regulations, allot the sums appropriated for such year pursuant to section 301 among the States on the basis of the relative population, financial need, and need for more effective prevention, treatment, and rehabilitation of alcohol abuse and alcoholism; except that no such allotment to any State (other than the Virgin Islands, American Samoa, Guam, and the Trust Territory of the Pacific Islands) for any fiscal year shall be less than $200,000.

(b) Any amount allotted to a State in a Fiscal year (other than the Virgin Islands, American Samoa, Guam, and the Trust Territory of the Pacific Islands) and remaining unobligated at the end of such year shall remain available to such State, for the purposes for which made, for the next fiscal year (and for such year only), and any such amount shall be in addition to the amounts allotted to such State for such purpose for such next fiscal year; except that any such amount, remaining unobligated at the end of the sixth month following the end of such year for which it was allotted, which the Secretary determines will remain unobligated by the close of such next fiscal year, may be reallotted by the Secretary, to be available for the purposes for which made until the close of such next fiscal year, to other States which have need therefor, on such basis as the Secretary deems equitable and consistent with the purposes of this part, and any amount so reallotted to a State shall be in addition to the amounts allotted and available to the States for the same period. Any amount allotted under subsection (a) to the Virgin Islands, American Samoa, Guam, or the Trust Territory of the Pacific Islands in a fiscal year and remaining unobligated at the end of such year shall remain available to it, for the purposes for which made, for the next two fiscal years (and for such years only), and any such amount shall be in addition to the amounts allotted to it for such purpose for each of such next two fiscal years; except that any such amount, remaining unobligated at the end of the first of such next two years, which the Secretary determines will remain unobligated at the close of the second of such next two years, may be reallotted by the Secretary, to be available for the purposes for which made until the close of the second of such next two years, to any other of such four States which have need therefor, on such basis as the Secretary deems equitable and consistent with the purposes of this part, and any amount so reallotted to a State shall be in addition to the amounts allotted and available to the State for the same period.

(c) At the request of any State, a portion of any allotment or allotments of such State under this part shall be available to pay that portion of the expenditures found necessary by the Secretary for the proper and efficient administration during such year of the State plan approved under this part, except that not more than 10 per centum of the total of the allotments of such State for a year, or $50,000, whichever is the least, shall be available for such purpose for such year.

(d) On the request of any State, the Secretary is authorized to arrange for the assignment of officers and employees of the Department or provide equipment or supplies in lieu of a portion of the allotment of such State. The allotment may be reduced by the fair market value of any equipment or supplies furnished to such State and by the amount of the pay, allowances, traveling expenses, and any other costs in connection with the detail of an officer or employee to the State. The amount by which such payments are so reduced shall be available for payment of such costs (including the costs of such equipment and supplies) by the Secretary, but shall for purposes of determining the allotment under section 302 (a), be deemed to have been paid to the State.

State Plans

Sec. 303. (a) Any State desiring to participate in this part shall submit a State plan for carrying out its purposes. Such plan must—

(1) designate a single State agency as the sole agency for the administration of the plan, or designate such agency as the sole agency for supervising the administration of the plan;

(2) contain satisfactory evidence that the State agency designated in accordance with paragraph (1) (hereafter in this section referred to as the "State agency") will have authority to carry out such plan in conformity with this part;

(3) provide for the designation of a State advisory council which shall include representatives of nongovernmental organizations, of groups to be served with attention to assuring representation of minority and poverty groups, and of public agencies concerned with the prevention and treatment of alcohol abuse and alcoholism, to consult with the State agency in carrying out the plan;

(4) set forth, in accordance with criteria established by the Secretary, a survey of need for the prevention and treatment of alcohol abuse and alcoholism, including a survey of the health facilities needed to provide services for alcohol abuse and alcoholism and a plan for the development and distribution of such facilities and programs throughout the State;

(5) provide such methods of administration of the State plan, including methods relating to the establishment and maintenance of personnel standards on a merit basis (except that the Secretary shall exercise no authority with respect to the selection, tenure of office, or compensation of any individual employed in accordance with such methods), as are found by the Secretary to be necessary for the proper and efficient operation of the plan;

(6) provide that the State agency will make such reports, in such form and containing such information, as the Secretary may from time to time reasonably require, and will keep such records and afford such access thereto as the Secretary may find necessary to assure the correctness and verification of such reports;

(7) provide that the Comptroller General of the United States or his duly authorized representatives shall have access for the purpose of audit and examination to the records specified in paragraph (6);

(8) provide that the State agency will from time to time, but not less often than annually, review its State plan and submit to the Secretary any modifications thereof which it considers necessary;

(9) provide reasonable assurance that Federal funds made available under this part for any period will be so used as to supplement and increase, to the extent feasible and practical, the level of State, local, and other non-Federal funds that would in the absence of such Federal funds be made available for the programs described in this part, and will in no event supplant such State, local, and other non-Federal funds;

(10) set forth, in accordance with criteria to be set by the Secretary, standards (including enforcement procedures and penalties) for (A) construction and licensing of public and private treatment facilities, and (B) for other community services or resources available to assist individuals to meet problems resulting from alcohol abuse; and

(11) contain such additional information and assurance as the Secretary may find necessary to carry out the provisions and purposes of this part.

(b) The Secretary shall approve any State plan and any modification thereof which complies with the provisions of subsection (a).

Special Grants for Implementation of the Uniform Alcoholism and Intoxication Treatment Act

Sec. 304. (a) To assist States which have adopted the basic provisions of the Uniform Alcoholism and Intoxication Treatment Act (hereinafter in this section referred to as the 'Uniform Act') to utilize fully the protections of the Uniform Act in their efforts to approach alcohol abuse and alcoholism from a community care standpoint, the Secretary, acting through the Institute, shall, during the period beginning July 1, 1974, and ending June 30, 1977, make grants to such States for the implementation of the Uniform Act. A grant under this section to any State may only be made for that State's costs (as determined in accordance with regulations which the Secretary shall promulgate not later than July 1, 1974) in implementing the Uniform Act for a period which does not exceed one year from the first day of the first month for which the grant is made. No State may receive more than three grants under this section.

(b) No grant may be made under this section unless an application therefor has been submitted to, and approved by, the Secretary. Such application shall be in such form, submitted in such manner, and contain such information as the Secretary shall by regulation prescribe. The Secretary may not approve an application of a State under this section unless he determines the following:

(1) The State and each of its political subdivisions are committed to the concept of care for alcoholism and alcohol abuse through community health and social service agencies, and, in accordance with the purposes of sections 1 and 19 of the Uniform Act, have repealed those portions of their criminal statutes and ordinances under which drunkenness is the gravamen of a petty criminal offense, such as loitering, vagrancy, or disturbing the peace.

(2) The laws of the State respecting acceptance of individuals into alcoholism and intoxication treatment programs are in accordance with the following standards of acceptance of individuals for such treatment (contained in section 10 of the Uniform Act):

(A) A patient shall, if possible, be treated on a voluntary rather than an involuntary basis.

(B) A patient shall be initially assigned or transferred to outpatient or intermediate treatment, unless he is found to require inpatient treatment.

(C) A person shall not be denied treatment solely because he has withdrawn from treatment against medical advice on a prior occasion or because he has relapsed after earlier treatment.

(D) An individualized treatment plan shall be prepared and maintained on a current basis for each patient.

(E) Provision shall be made for a continuum of coordinated treatment services so that a person who leaves a facility or a form of treatment will have available and utilize other appropriate treatment.

(3) The laws of the State respecting involuntary commitment of alcoholics are consistent with the provisions of section 14 of the Uniform Act which protect individual rights.

(4) The application of the State contains such assurances as the Secretary may require to carry out the purposes of this section.

For purposes of subsection (a), the term "basic provisions of the Uniform Alcoholism and Intoxication Treatment Act" shall not in the case of a State which has a State plan approved under section 303 include any provision of the Uniform Act respecting the organization of such State's treatment programs (as defined in the Uniform Act) which are inconsistent with the requirements of such State plan.

(c) The amount of any grant under this section to any State for any fiscal year may not exceed the sum of $100,000 and an amount equal to 10 per centum of the allotment of such State for such fiscal year under section 302 of this Act. Payments under grants under this section may be made in advance or by way of reimbursement, and at such intervals and on such conditions as the Secretary finds necessary.

(d) For the purpose of making payments under grants under this section, there are authorized to be appropriated $13,000,000 for the fiscal year ending June 30, 1975, and for each of the next two fiscal years.

Part B—Project Grants and Contracts

Grants and Contracts for the Prevention and Treatment of Alcohol Abuse and Alcoholism

Sec. 311. (a) The Secretary, acting through the Institute, may make grants to public and nonprofit private entities and may enter into contracts with public and private entities and with individuals—

(1) to conduct demonstration, service, and evaluation projects,

(2) to provide education and training,

(3) to provide programs and services in cooperation with schools, courts, penal institutions, and other public agencies, and

(4) to provide counseling and education activities on an individual or community basis,

for the prevention and treatment of alcohol abuse and alcoholism and for the rehabilitation of alcohol abusers and alcoholics.

(b) Projects and programs for which grants and contracts are made under this section shall (1) whenever possible, be community based, seek to insure care of good quality in general community care facilities and under health insurance plans, and be integrated with, and provide for the active participation of, a wide range of public and nongovernmental agencies, organizations, institutions, and individuals; and (2) where appropriate utilize existing community resources (including community mental health centers).

(c) (1) In administering this section, the Secretary shall require coordination of all applications for projects and programs in a State.

(2) Each applicant from within a State, upon filing its application with the Secretary for a grant or contract under this section, shall submit a copy of its application for review by the State agency designated under section 303 of this Act, if such designation has been made. Such State agency shall be given not more than thirty days from the date of receipt of the application to submit to the Secretary, in writing, an evaluation of the project or program set forth in the application. Such evaluation shall include comments on the relationship to the project to other projects and programs pending and approved and to the State comprehensive plan for treatment and prevention of alcohol abuse and alcoholism under section 303. The State shall furnish the applicant a copy of any such evaluation.

(3) Approval of any application for a grant or contract by the Secretary, including the earmarking of financial assistance for a program or project, may be granted only if the application substantially meets a set of criteria established by the Secretary that—

(A) provides that the projects and programs for which assistance under this section is sought will be substantially administered by or under the supervision of the applicant;

(B) provides for such methods of administration as are necessary for the proper and efficient operation of such programs and projects;

(C) provides for such fiscal control and fund accounting procedures as may be necessary to assure proper disbursement of and accounting for Federal funds paid to the applicant; and

(D) provides reasonable assurance that Federal funds made available under this section for any period will be so used as to supplement and increase, to the extent feasible and practical, the level of State, local, and other non-Federal funds that would in the absence of such Federal funds be made available for the projects and programs described in this section, and will in no event supplant such State, local, and other non-Federal funds.

(d) To make payments under grants and contracts under this section, there are authorized to be appropriated $80,000,000 for the fiscal year ending June 30, 1975, and $95,000,000 for the fiscal year ending June 30, 1976.

Part C—Admission to Hospitals

Admission of Alcohol Abusers and Alcoholics to Private and Public Hospitals

Sec. 321. (a) Alcohol abusers and alcoholics who are suffering from medical conditions shall not be discriminated against in admission or treatment, solely because of their alcohol abuse or alcoholism, by any private or public general hospital which receives support in any form from any program supported in whole or in part by funds appropriated to any Federal department or agency.

(b) (1) The Secretary is authorized to make regulations for the enforcement of the policy of subsection (a) with respect to the admission and treatment of alcohol abusers and alcoholics in hospitals which receive support of any kind from any program administered by the Secretary. Such regulations shall include procedures for determining (after opportunity for a hearing if requested) if a violation of subsection (a) has occurred, notification of failure to comply with such subsection, and opportunity for a violator to comply with such subsection. If the Secretary determines that a hospital subject to such regulations has violated subsection (a) and such violation continues after an opportunity has been afforded for compliance, the Secretary may suspend or revoke, after opportunity for a hearing, all or part of any support of any kind received by such hospital from any program administered by the Secretary. The Secretary may consult with the officials responsible for the administration of any other Federal program from which such hospital receives support of any kind, with respect to the suspension or revocation of such other Federal support for such hospital.

(2) The Administrator of Veterans' Affairs, through the Chief Medical Director, shall, to the maximum feasible extent consistent with their responsibilities under title 38, United States Code, prescribe regulations making applicable the regulations prescribed by the Secretary under paragraph (1) of this subsection to the provision of hospital care, nursing home care, domiciliary care, and medical services under such title 38 to veterans suffering from alcohol abuse or alcoholism. In prescribing and implementing regulations pursuant to this paragraph, the Administrator shall, from time to time, consult with the Secretary in order to achieve the maximum possible coordination of the regulations, and the implementation thereof, which they each prescribe.

Part D—General

Comprehensive State Health Plans
Sec. 331. Section 314 (d) (2) of the Public Health Service Act is amended—

(1) by striking out "and" at the end of subparagraph (J);

(2) by striking out the period at the end of subparagraph (K) and inserting in lieu thereof "; and"; and

(3) by adding after subparagraph (K) the following new subparagraph;

"(L) provide for services for the prevention and treatment of alcohol abuse and alcoholism, commensurate with the extent of the problem."

Specialized Facilities
Sec. 332. Section 243 (a) of the Community Health Centers Act is amended (1) by inserting "or leasing" after "construction" and (2) by inserting "facilities for emergency medical services, intermediate care services, or outpatient services, and "immediately before "posthospitalization treatment facilities."

Confidentiality of Records
Sec. 333 (a) Records of the identity, diagnosis, prognosis, or treatment of any patient which are maintained in connection with the performance of any program or activity relating to alcoholism or alcohol abuse education, training, treatment, rehabilitation, or research, which is conducted, regulated, or directly or indirectly assisted by any department or agency of the United States shall, except as provided in subsection (e), be confidential and be disclosed only for the purposes and under the circumstances expressly authorized under subsection (b) of this section.

(b) (1) The content of any record referred to in subsection (a) may be disclosed in accordance with the prior written consent of the patient with respect to whom such record is maintained, but only to such extent, under such circumstances, and for such purposes as may be allowed under regulations prescribed pursuant to subsection (g).

(2) Whether or not the patient, with respect to whom any given record referred to in subsection (a) of this section is maintained, gives his written consent, the content of such record may be disclosed as follows:

(A) To medical personnel to the extent necessary to meet a bona fide medical emergency.

(B) To qualified personnel for the purpose of conducting scientific research, management audits, financial audits, or program evaluation, but such personnel may not identify, directly or indirectly, any individual patient in any report of such research, audit, or evaluation, or otherwise disclose patient identities in any manner.

(C) If authorized by an appropriate order of a court of competent jurisdiction granted after application showing good cause therefore. In assessing good cause the court shall weigh the public interest and the need for disclosure against the injury to the patient, to the physician-patient relationship, and to the treatment services. Upon the granting of such order, the court, in determining the extent to which any disclosure of all or any part of any record is necessary, shall impose appropriate safeguards against unauthorized disclosure.

(c) Except as authorized by a court order granted under subsection (b) (2) (C) of this section, no record referred to in subsection (a) may be used to initiate or substantiate any criminal charges against a patient or to conduct any investigation of a patient.

(d) The prohibitions of this section continue to apply to records concerning any individual who has been a patient, irrespective of whether or when he ceases to be a patient.

(e) The prohibitions of this section do not apply to any interchange of records—

(1) within the Armed Forces or within those components of the Veterans' Administration furnishing health care to veterans, or

(2) between such components and the Armed Forces.

(f) Any person who violates any provision of this section or any regulation issued pursuant to this section shall be fined not more than $500 in the case of a first offense, and not more than $5,000 in the case of each subsequent offense.

(g) Except as provided in subsection (h) of this section, the Secretary shall prescribe regulations to carry out the purposes of this section. These regulations may contain such definitions, and may provide for such safeguards and procedures, including procedures and criteria for the issuance and scope of orders under subsection (b) (2) (C), as in the judgment of the Secretary are necessary or proper to effectuate the purposes of this section, to prevent circumvention or evasion thereof, or to facilitate compliance therewith.

(h) The Administrator of Veterans' Affairs, through the Chief Medical Director, shall, to the maximum feasible extent consistent with their responsibilities under title 38, United States Code, prescribe regulations making applicable the regulations prescribed by the Secretary under subsection (g) of this section to records maintained in connection with the provision of hospital care, nursing home care, domiciliary care, and medical services under such title 38 to veterans suffering from alcohol abuse or alcoholism. In prescribing and implementing regulations pursuant to this subsection, the Administrator shall, from time to time, consult with the Secretary in order to achieve the maximum possible coordination of the regulations, and the implementation thereof, which they each prescribe.

Title IV—The National Advisory Council on Alcohol Abuse and Alcoholism

Establishment of Council

Sec. 401. (a) Section 217 (a) of the Public Health Service Act is amended—

(1) in the first sentence thereof, by inserting "the National Advisory Council on Alcohol Abuse and Alcoholism," immediately after "the National Advisory Mental Health Council,";

(2) in the second sentence thereof, by (A) inserting "the National Advisory Council on Alcoholic Abuse and Alcoholism," immediately after "the National Advisory Mental Health Council,", and (B) inserting "alcohol abuse and alcoholism," immediately after "psychiatric disorders,"; and

(3) in the fourth sentence, (A) by inserting "(other than the members of the National Advisory Council on Alcohol Abuse and Alcoholism)" after "the terms of the members"; (B) by striking out "and" before"(2)"; and (C) by striking out the period at the end and inserting a semicolon and "and (3) the terms of the members of the National Council on Alcohol Abuse and Alcoholism first taking office after the date of enactment of this clause, shall expire as follows: Three shall expire four years after such date, three shall expire three years after such date, three shall expire two years after such date, and three shall expire one year after such date, as designated by the Secretary at the time of appointment."

(b) Section 217 (b) of such Act is amended, in the second sentence thereof, by inserting "alcohol abuse and alcoholism," immediately after "mental health,".

(c) Section 217 of such Act is further amended by adding at the end thereof the following new subsection:

"(d) The National Advisory Council on Alcohol Abuse and Alcoholism shall advise, consult with, and make recommendations to, the Secretary on matters relating to the activities and functions of the Secretary in the field of alcohol abuse and alcoholism. The Council is authorized (1) to review research projects or programs submitted to or initiated by it in the field of alcohol abuse and alcoholism and recommend to the Secretary any such projects which it believes show promise of making valuable contributions to human knowledge with respect to the cause, prevention, or methods of diagnosis and treatment of alcohol abuse and alcoholism, and (2) to collect information as to studies being carried on in the field of alcohol abuse and alcoholism and, with the approval of the Secretary, make available such information through appropriate publications for the benefit of health and welfare agencies or organizations (public or private) or physicians or any other scientists, and for the information of the general public. The Council is also authorized to recommend to the Secretary, for acceptance pursuant to section 501 of this Act, conditional gifts for work in the field of alcohol abuse and alcoholism; and the Secretary shall recommend acceptance of any such gifts only after consultation with the Council."

Approval by Council of Certain Grants Under Part C of Community Mental Health Centers Act

Sec. 402. Section 266 of the Community Mental Health Centers Act is amended (1) by inserting "(Other than part C thereof)" immediately after "this title", and (2) by adding immediately after the period the following: "Grants under part C of this title for such costs may be made only upon recommendation of the National Advisory Council on Alcohol Abuse and Alcoholism established by such section."

Title V—General

Sec. 501. If any section, provision, or term of this Act is adjudged invalid for any reason, such judgment shall not affect, impair, or invalidate any other section, provision, or term of this Act, and the remaining sections, provisions, and terms shall be and remain in full force and effect.

Sec. 502. (a) Each recipient of assistance under this Act pursuant to grants or contracts entered into under other than competitive bidding procedures shall keep such records as the Secretary shall prescribe, including records which fully disclose the amount and disposition by such recipient of the proceeds of such grant or contract, the total cost of the project or undertaking in connection with which such grant or contract is given or used, and the amount of that portion of the cost of the project or undertaking supplied by other sources, and such other records as will facilitate an effective audit.

(b) The Secretary and Comptroller General of the United States, or any of their duly authorized representatives, shall have access for the purpose of audit and examination to any books, documents, papers, and records of such recipients that are pertinent to the grants or contracts entered into under the provisions of this Act under other than competitive bidding procedures.

Sec. 503. Payments under this Act may be made in advance or by way of reimbursement and in such installments as the Secretary may determine.

Appendix D

GOVERNMENT POLICY AND THE PROBLEM OF ALCOHOLISM

Government Policy and the Problem of Alcoholism

A Report of the
Section on Drug and Alcohol Abuse
of the
Department of Psychiatry
of the
Medical College of Pennsylvania
at
Eastern Pennsylvania Psychiatric Institute

Prepared by:
Frederick B. Glaser, M.D., Chief
Section on Drug and Alcohol Abuse

Acknowledgements

Many persons helped in the preparation of this report. The support of the entire staff of the Section on Drug and Alcohol Abuse was critical. Dr. Richard Horman suggested its preparation and made many helpful suggestions during its completion. Dr. Robert E. Popham of the Addiction Research Foundation in Toronto, Canada, and Mark Keller of the Rutgers Center of Alcohol Studies gave both their time and their materials to assist us. The libraries at Eastern Pennsylvania Psychiatric Institute and the Medical College of Pennsylvania were most helpful. Mary Connelly typed the manuscript. A particular expression of thanks goes to Mrs. Stephanie Greenburg, research assistant, whose cheerful and assiduous bibliographic assistance provided most of the necessary materials. Responsibility for the defects of the report rests exclusively with its preparer.

F.B.G.
December 5th, 1973

Table of Contents

Appendices:*

A. Correspondence between Richard E. Horman, Ph.D., executive Director, Governor's Council on Drug and Alcohol Abuse, and Frederick B. Glaser, M.D., chief, section on Drug and Alcohol Abuse of the Department of Psychiatry of the Medical College of Pennsylvania at Eastern Pennsylvania Psychiatric Institute, relative to the preparation of a report on government policy and the problem of alcoholism.
B. Popham, Robert E., Wolfgang Schmidt, and Jan deLint. The prevention of alcoholism: epidemiological studies of the effects of government control measures. Manuscript. To be published in: Ewing, J.A., and Rouse, B.A. (eds.): *Law and Drinking Behavior,* Chapel Hill, University of North Carolina Press. Manuscript originally received September 7, 1973. Permission given for limited distribution by telephone November 5, 1973.
C. Letter from Mark Keller, editor, *Quarterly Journal of Studies on Alcohol,* 12 November 1973.
D. Table indicating mechanisms utilized by states dedicating liquor revenues to alcoholism programs.
E. Correspondence from the South Carolina Commission on Alcoholism relative to that state's "mini-bottle legislation," together with copies of the relevant acts of the South Carolina legislature.

* The appendices were included in the original report but are not reproduced here.

Summary and Conclusions

At the request of Richard E. Horman, Ph.D., executive director of the Governor's Council on Drug and Alcohol Abuse, the Section on Drug and Alcohol Abuse of the Department of Psychiatry of the Medical College of Pennsylvania at Eastern Pennsylvania Psychiatric Institute has examined the literature on the relationship between government policy and the problem of alcoholism. The following conclusions were drawn from this study.

1. Many different government policies have been framed over a long period of time in an effort to control the problem of alcoholism.
2. Those government policies in use in the United States at present, including the state monopoly system in Pennsylvania, are largely ineffective in controlling alcoholism.
3. Some effective measures which have been used in the past in the United States are no longer feasible, or are not feasible in Pennsylvania.
4. One potentially effective measure which has not yet been used in the United States or in Pennsylvania is the control of alcoholism by government control of the price of alcohol. There is a large body of empirical evidence which attributes the progressive increase in alcoholism to the progressive decline in the price of alcohol. This suggests that raising the price of alcohol would arrest and/or reverse the increase of alcoholism.
5. Termination of the state liquor monopoly in Pennsylvania with dispersal of the retail function into private hands is *not* recommended for the following reasons:
   a. It would create a large and politically powerful vested interest group which would lobby effectively for low alcohol prices. The activities of this group would very likely preclude the use of the price mechanism to control alcoholism.
   b. It would increase the incidence of alcoholism by lowering the price of alcohol. Whatever short-term advantages might be gained in terms of increased tax revenues would subsequently be lost, perhaps several times over, through the increased costs accruing to alcoholism and its complications.
6. Retention of the state liquor monopoly and an attempt to control alcoholism by raising the price of alcoholic beverages relative to disposable income presents many problems. Among the measures which could be taken to ameliorate these problems are effective public education regarding the costs and hazards of alcoholism, dedication of the revenues gained by the price increase to the combatting of alcoholism, and the coordination of an interstate or regional approach to the problem.
7. The Section on Drug and Alcohol Abuse will continue to keep the

Governor's Council on Drug and Alcohol Abuse informed of relevant advances in alcoholism research which bear upon this problem.

Respectfully Submitted,

Frederick B. Glaser, M.D., Chief
for the
Section on Drug and Alcohol Abuse

Government Policy and the Problem of Alcoholism

Introduction.

This report is written against a background of governmental deliberations on the fate of the state liquor monopoly in Pennsylvania. Its efficient cause was a request from Richard E. Horman, Ph.D., executive director of the Governor's Council on Drug and Alcohol Abuse. In his letter of September 21, 1973 addressed to Frederick B. Glaser, M.D., chief of the Section on Drug and Alcohol Abuse of the Medical College of Pennsylvania, Dr. Horman stated in part:

> *I would like to request that your staff assemble for the Governor such information as can be found concerning the effect or lack of effect of state monopolies on liquor or other information concerning the casual factors in alcoholism as it relates to the availability of substance.*

Because the correspondence between Dr. Horman and Dr. Glaser contains much material relevant to this report but not otherwise contained in it, the letters themselves will be included among the appended materials (see Appendix A). The staff of the SDAA have endeavored to comply with Dr. Horman's directive. The relevant literature in the field has been searched out through computerized search systems (e.g. MEDLINE), through published bibliographies, and through consultation with knowledgeable individuals. Expert groups of researchers in the field of alcoholism have also been consulted, in particular the Addiction Research Foundation of Toronto, Canada, and the Rutgers Center of Alcohol Studies in New Brunswick, New Jersey. Written and telephone contact has been made with many state and national agencies in the field, most of whom were extremely helpful.* At the same time, in accordance with Dr. Horman's wishes, the investigation has been kept entirely confidential.

Critically reviewed and digested, the information which has been gathered is here summarized. The present report must be considered incomplete. This is due largely to the time constraints under which it has been prepared and the considerable difficulty in assembling materials on this particular topic. There are very few sources, and those which exist are particularly hard to get. Many of them, such as the extensive literature on the pre-revolutionary Russian state alcohol

* A notable exception to this was the Liquor Control Board of the Commonwealth of Pennsylvania, which supplied no material of any kind useful in the preparation of this report, in spite of requests by SDAA staff.

monopoly, exist only in languages other than English. Several additional sources are en route to the SDAA, but have not arrived in time for this report.

Nevertheless it is our belief that the data are reasonably complete and that additional data are unlikely to alter the general outlines of our conclusions. Therefore, a report at this point in time seems warranted, though further work will be done. The report will commence with a general survey of governmental policies on controlling the sale of alcohol and their effects on the incidence of alcoholism. This will lead to a discussion of four highly correlated variables which might form the basis of a variety of control which has not as yet been attempted. These four variables are the incidence of alcoholism, the incidence of deaths due to cirrhosis of the liver, the per capita consumption of alcohol, and the price of alcohol. The paper will conclude with a discussion of various aspects of government control of the alcohol price mechanism.

Government Control of the Sale of Alcohol: The Monopoly System

Contrary to our belief when research on this project was begun, government control over the sale of alcohol is neither new, nor specifically American, nor limited in our own history to Prohibition and its aftermath. For example, the Russian government regulated the sale of alcohol as far back as the time of Tsar Boris Goudounof (1598-1601) and throughout the 19th century made a determined effort in this direction. It went by the boards for a time but was reintroduced in 1895, at first in a few provinces and subsequently, when it appeared to be successful, into the whole Empire (1). Sweden's "Gothenburg" and "Bratt" systems of control, in widespread use throughout the 19th century, served as a model for the Canadian provinces (2), and Canada in turn served as a model for many American state plans following the repeal of Prohibition. A large group of the states which currently have monopoly systems lie along the Canadian border (3) and in some states the evidence of Canadian influence is quite direct. Thus, prior to the passage of the state monopoly legislation in Pennsylvania, Governor Gifford Pinchot sent at least four state officials to study the state control systems in Ontario and Quebec (4, p. 8). Even in Pennsylvania, the legislation passed in 1933 had its ancestor in the Brooks law, "a statute which served as the keystone of Pennsylvania liquor control from 1887 until Prohibition became effective in 1920" (4, p. 7).

Pennsylvania does, however, have the honor of being the first of the United States to implement a state liquor monopoly in the post-Prohibition period. The stores which first opened for business on Tuesday, January 2, 1934 will soon pass their 40th anniversary. Other states, in setting up their control systems, came to learn from us (5). The Commonwealth's Liquor Control Board was said to be, at least at one time, the largest purchaser of liquor in the world. For example, in the single month of December 1947, the 575 state stores operating in Pennsylvania sold 963,175 cases of liquor. Since 1,500 cases are equivalent to one carload, "Pennsylvania's liquor train for that month ... totalled 642 cars" (4, p. 24).

Sixteen other states have set up monopoly systems roughly similar to that in Pennsylvania, at least in the sense that both retail and wholesale control is exerted. A 17th state, Wyoming, operates in the wholesale area only; and Mississippi is dry. Taken collectively, these states have tried a wide variety of administrative arrangements (2, 6, 7) over a long time. One is therefore entitled to hope that something definitive might have been learned from this collective experience. But with a very few exceptions, this is a vain hope. Ten years ago, the Moreland Commission of the State of New York asked the Rutgers Center of Alcohol Studies to provide them with an answer to the question: "Do controls over the selling of alcoholic beverages induce temperate use of such beverages?" In response, the Rutgers group made two general points:

> *... one, there are almost no studies of this relationship for any American jurisdiction; two, the sorts of record(s) and information necessary for sufficient answers are either (a) quite inadequate or (b) have been collected or prepared for purposes so different from that of answering this or any related question that validated, definitive statements are just not available. (3, p. 7)*

So far as we are aware, that statement still stands. In the 10 years which have elapsed since it was written, no definitive studies have been made which would provide the answers. As we shall see, this did not prevent the Rutgers group from reaching some tentative conclusions, nor shall it prevent us. But it must be recognized that any such conclusions *are* tentative. The astonishing fact remains that despite 40 years' experience and the use of many and varied control systems, we really do not know what has happened. This is but one specific example of the general lack of any research upon the effects of governmental policies (8).

Proceeding now in a somewhat more gingerly manner, and not being upon ground which is as solid as one might wish, we may cautiously conclude that existing data indicate that governmental control of the sale of alcohol has failed to have any effect upon the incidence of alcoholism. The incidence of alcoholism has risen in both monopoly and non-monopoly states. For example, data from 1964 indicate no statistically significant differences between monopoly and license states in such parameters as the consumption of wine, spirits, beer, or total alcohol or in mortality rates from liver cirrhosis, a measure closely correlated with the incidence of alcoholism (9, Table 1). This is broadly representative of much other data, further adumbrated by the Rutgers group and summarized by them as follows:

(1) Existing differences in the commercial controls utilized by different states to control the direct problems of alcohol do not seem to produce consistent or significant differences in the reported occurrence of those problems.

(2) Where differences in the reported occurrences of direct problems of alcohol do appear among the jurisdictions with differing systems of commercial control, they give every indication of being the result of factors other than those of the commercial control system. (3, pp. 7-8)

The Failure of the Monopoly System: Reasons

Why is this so? A brief examination of reasons may be helpful in planning for the future. First, it must be said that if the reduction of alcoholism was one of the purposes of the legislation which established state liquor monopolies, explicit statements of this purpose are noticeably absent from both the legislation and from related materials. Thus there is no mention of alcoholism as a problem either in the eight reasons given by Governor Pinchot for the introduction of the monopoly system in Pennsylvania (4, p. 8) or in the five reasons given by Mr. Smith for its introduction in New Hampshire (5). Perhaps the conceptualization of alcoholism at that time was rudimentary. One gathers it was believed that the ordinary man, left to his own devices, would automatically either avoid alcohol or would drink moderately. He would only develop a problem with alcohol if enticed into excess, either by the many amenities of the saloon or by the desire of the publican for profit. The very first point in Governor Pinchot's program was "the saloon must not come back" (4, p. 8) while Smith sees the first object of the state store as "the satisfaction of a normal, unstimulated demand for liquor" (5). There is much material here for further historical investigation. But one of the reasons the monopoly system has not controlled alcoholism may be that the control of alcoholism was not intended or perhaps even considered.

Even with respect to carrying out the clearly expressed intent of its framers the laws generally failed. The saloon is an example. Historically the austere ambience of the Pennsylvania state store is a direct consequence of the attempt to avoid the trappings of the old saloon. At first the state stores were permitted to display wares in their windows, but a governor's directive put a stop to this: it was too reminiscent of the saloon. Governor Pinchot, who superintended the passage of the initial legislation, was "an avowed dry who twice had campaigned for governor on a bone-dry platform. Moreover, for about 10 years he had sat on the State Board of Trustees of the Anti-Saloon League" (4, p. 9). No wonder his first item of priority was the prohibition of the saloon. Yet the Pennsylvania legislation, for all that, permitted the licensing of businesses for the on-premises consumption of liquor (other states, as we shall see, did not). The result was that in Pennsylvania,

> *... the expressed hope that the saloon would never return has not been realized. The name is somewhat forgotten, but the establishment still exists. At times it is called a tavern and at others a tap room. It must be able to produce some kind of food to pass the inspection of enforcement officers. And in many cases it has lost its swinging doors. But it is still the twin brother of the pre-prohibition saloon. (4, p. 69)*

If the omission of control over on-premises consumption was one reason for the failure of the monopoly law to control alcoholism, its failure to control alcoholic beverages other than spiritous liquors was certainly another. It has been widely argued that alcoholism is due to the consumption of liquor, and that beer and wine, the "beverages of moderation," are exempt from responsibility. The term "wino" should be enough to vitiate this argument, but there are more solid grounds, summarized by the Canadian researchers (9, pp. 10-12). Total alcohol consumed is the significant factor, and it can be gotten through any alcohol-containing beverage; many alcoholics use beer and wine as their drink of preference. With this in mind it is relevant that the distribution of beer was permitted in Pennsylvania from the very beginning and was not controlled under the monopoly system. Indeed, in the initial legislation the issuance of beer distribution licenses was the responsibility of county officials, though it later reverted to the Board. In permitting beer distribution the Pennsylvania lawmakers may have been following a national precedent. On April 7, 1933 the U.S. congress legalized the distribution of beer which contained 3.2% alcohol by weight. Pennsylvania did the same on May 3rd, while Prohibition was not repealed until December 5 of that year (see reference 4 for these points).

Another among the failures of this legislation with respect to the control of alcoholism was its failure to deal with the profit motive. This failure was not due to lack of recognition. The crucial importance of the profit motive had been recognized at least as early as 1895, when the Russians hoped their state monopoly would "... free (the peasants) ... from exploitation by the publicans, for whom drunkenness and debauch were the best sources of income" (1,p.3). Governor Pinchot's third point was that "private profit from liquor must be reduced to the minimum" (4, p.8). Landis quotes a 1933 report which studied liquor control systems in 12 countries, including the United States and Canada, as follows:

> *... we firmly believe that any system of control which does not attack the private profit motive in the retail sale of spirits is merely touching the problem at its fringe. Unless we eliminate the incentive behind the stimulation of sales, we have not dug to the root of the difficulty, and the weeds of abuse will thrive no matter how we hack.*

But there is no particular reason for preferring public profit to private profit. It is still the profit motive which drives up the sales, the only difference being that it is the state's general fund which benefits and not the purse of an individual. If there is a profit to be made, sales will be pushed, whether individual or collective profits are involved. Pennsylvania provides an excellent example. Its liquor control board issued the following announcement a few days before the stores opened for business for the first time:

> *These are your stores. They are operated by your state government. Profits from their operations are paid only into your state treasury to meet appropriations for relief and pensions to the blind and aged. Every Pennsylvanian may feel justly proud of the principles back of these state-operated stores. Every loyal citizen, by patronage and cooperation, will assist in their success (4, p.13).*

As McGeary remarked, "To a host of disapproving ears, this statement sounded as if the state believed that citizens had a patriotic duty to drink" (4, p.13). It is not surprising. The state stores were founded during the depths of the Depression, and one of the major motives behind their establishment was to provide much-needed revenue to defray the expenses of that economic misfortune. This was true on the federal level as well. An anonymous contributor to the *Harvard Law Review* in 1933 held that the legal basis upon which the United States government taxed state liquor monopolies was invalid. However, he also believed it would be upheld in the courts if tested at that time, because of "the crying need of the general government for immediate revenue. It is common knowledge that the United States is relying heavily upon liquor taxes to support the lion's share of the expensive emergency relief program" (10, p.324).

Thus, rather than dealing decisively with the profit motive in alcohol sales, all the monopoly legislation did was to substitute public profit for private profit. In a few states, such as Michigan, a commission was actually built into the state monopoly (6, p.580) to encourage sales. And it was a big business. In 1946 the gross sales of the 16 state monopoly systems amounted to over $2.5 billion (7), while in the same year the Commonwealth of Pennsylvania netted $31.7 million from sales alone, some six times the net profit in the first year of operation (4, p.64). Not only did the profit motive remain under the monopoly system, but it may well have been enhanced. There is a good deal of evidence that with a monopoly system, a state can extract more profit than under a license system (4, 11-13) while still offering liquor to the consumer at a slightly lower cost. According to Simon (13) this is due to three things: the "monopsonistic" purchasing of liquor by monopoly states under the so-called "Des Moines agreement," according to which monopoly states are guaranteed a price no higher than the lowest price to wholesalers in private-license states; lower operating costs, due to the operation of fewer outlets for shorter hours; and the somewhat larger margins of private profit. Simon concludes that "by any measure, the treasuries of monopoly states net much more money from the liquor trade carried on within their borders than do private license states" (13, p.193).

Virtually all of the money thus earned goes directly into the general fund of the state, and for the most part this has been so from the very beginning. Perhaps this fact, more than anything else, indicates the power of the profit motive even in the monopoly system. As Landis points out, the profits are never used to reduce the price of alcohol and thereby liquidate themselves, as would perhaps be the case if control were the primary goal of the system. (As we shall have occasion to see, Landis' notion may be correct, but reduction of price would likely have the opposite effect from what he intended). Thus the profit motive still assists in the promotion of alcohol sales and has not been eliminated by monopoly legislation; it may, indeed, have assumed an even greater importance.

To sum up this section of the report, it is not surprising to find that, in general, government control measures have failed to decrease the incidence of alcoholism. There is little indication that this is what they were intended to do at the time they were framed, perhaps because of naive views of the nature and etiology of that condition. In spite of explicit intentions to the contrary, the saloon was not eliminated but simply called something else. Failure to recognize that beer and wine were implicated in alcoholism as well as the "ardent spirits" left them essentially without control. Shifting from private profit to public profit may have salved a few consciences and quieted others, but it still left the profit motive critically operative in alcoholism sales. These shortcomings may have been what E. M. Jellinek, the father of modern alcoholism research, had in mind when he commented that "In fairness, it must be said that a true monopoly system has not been tried out" (14, p.27).

Lessons from the Monopoly System

Every cloud, one supposes, has a silver lining. Despite the pessimistic conclusions developed by the Rutgers people for the Moreland Commission (see above, p.5), some few positive things have been observed. They may indicate that the possibility of developing effective government policies on the sale of alcohol which might limit the incidence of alcoholism are not entirely beyond question. The authors of the Rutgers survey were careful to leave the door open. In their summary and conclusions they observed that their findings related only to the control systems then being employed in the United States, and specifically said that their survey "does not relate to any possible sales control system" (3, p.53).

One sales control system not being used at the time of the survey was the complete suppression of sales, that is, Prohibition. That era of our national life is generally believed to have been so unfortunate that it is little examined and, when it is, is usually blamed for the emergence of organized crime. However, organized crime was present long before Prohibition went into effect. Although it utilized Prohibition as a vehicel for self-aggrandisement, it is a moot point whether in the absence of Prohibition organized crime would not have found an alternative vehicle which would have served equally well. And of course it has now long survived the demise of Prohibition. Beyond this, Canada, which had a more prolonged experience with Prohibition, did not develop an organized crime apparatus similar to that in the United States. Thus the hypothesis that organized crime in the United States resulted directly from Prohibition requires further investigation.

Because of the great interest in the crime question, other questions about the era are infrequently asked. One possible question would relate to the incidence of alcoholism during Prohibition. E. M. Jellinek felt that Prohibition had a marked impact on alcoholism. In a classic paper, he presented convincing data which indicated that both the per capita consumption of alcohol and the rate of alcoholism declined considerably during Prohibition (14). Doubtless this news will not raise much enthusiasm for the re-introduction of the Eighteenth Amendment. But it does indicate that at least some governmental control measures may have been effective against alcoholism.

Partial prohibition may also be effective. At the time of the Moreland Commission report, there were 12 states which prohibited on-premises sales, five of which were also monopoly states. That is, in these 12 states one could not purchase liquor by the drink. One could buy only from a package store, and, in five instances, only from a state-owned package store. This arrangement bears some similarity to the Russian monopoly system, wherein the rationale was that "the consumption of spiritous drinks at home, under the watchful eye of the family, is a certain guarantee for a more moderate consumption of alcoholic beverages" (1, p.3). Be that as it may, the prohibition of on-premises consumption is at least a more rigorous system of control than in Pennsylvania. The Moreland Commission report notes that 10 of the 12 states with this prohibition were to be found among the 13 states with the lowest per capita consumption of distilled spirits. The Commission is quite uncomfortable with this data and repeatedly attempts to explain it away. But it succeeds only in showing that while such a system *tends* to succeed, it does not necessarily succeed. Even though this partial expedient is less rigorous than total Prohibition, it would not seem a reasonable solution for Pennsylvania's current situation. Once certain steps have been taken it is hard to retrace them. But again, the point is that not *all* government control methods have been totally inefficacious.

Government control of the advertising of alcohol is also of interest. While there is no hard evidence favoring its efficacy it is generally conceded to have been effective. Certainly the widespread advertising of alcohol products would not tend to diminish the consumption of alcohol. As summarized by Archibald,

> *...there is no reason to believe that alcoholic beverages differ in any way from any other consumer goods. Volume and pattern of alcohol sales are affected by advertising just as are sales of television sets or cars. There seems to be no question, judging in part from the industry's own use of the media, that advertising—particularly by television—exerts a powerful influence over drinking styles and particularly over the developing habits of young people. (23, pp. 12-13).*

But rules on advertising practices vary widely. This variability gave rise to what is surely one of the more felicitous remarks in the whole of the alcoholism literature:

> *New York is one of the few states which expressly approve the use of Santa Claus in liquor advertising, on the ground that "he's not actually a saint, but a character of fiction, not a biblical character, but merely a symbol of happiness and good cheer"—a regulation which reveals that the commission's ignorance of church history is matched only by its misunderstanding of the functions of advertising control. (6, pp.568-69)*

The Price Mechanism as a Possible Means of Control

Finally, alcoholism research has suggested a possible method of control exercised by government that has not been attempted in North America, but has met with considerable success elsewhere (e.g. Finland). This is the manipulation of the price structure of alcohol to control its use. By deliberate increase of the price of alcohol through taxation and/or other means, it is felt that a profound effect can be exercised on the incidence of alcoholism. The argument has been pressed mainly by Canadian researchers (9, 15). It depends upon two general observations and upon a series of correlations between factors which constitute a plausible etiologic chain. The factors will be discussed below in some detail. The general observations are, first, that there is a rather remarkable inverse correlation between the price of alcohol and alcohol consumption. The greater the percentage of his available income that a man must spend to purchase a given amount of alcohol, the less likely he is to become an alcoholic. (See especially 9, Table 5). Second, in at least some Western jurisdictions the opposite has been happening, namely, there has been a steady decline in the price of alcohol relative to disposable income, while at the same time alcoholism has been increasing (see especially 9, Figure 1). So well are the arguments concerning this set out in an as yet unpublished paper by Robert Popham and his associates that we are including it as an appendix to this report, and urge that it be most carefully studied (see Appendix B). We are deeply grateful to Mr. Popham for giving us his permission to distribute the paper prior to publication.

In order to understand this very important argument, the interrelationship between four important factors will be discussed. This material is intended as a supplement to the paper of Popham *et al.,* and is not a substitute for its careful perusal. Discussing the four factors will also allow us to introduce some material of importance to Pennsylvania. The four factors to be discussed are: the incidence of alcoholism; the incidence of death from cirrhosis of the liver; the per capita consumption of alcohol; and the price of alcohol.

Because of the difficulty and expense of making a direct determination of the incidence of alcoholism through a field study with numerous interviews or by other means, an indirect estimate of prevalence estimation has long been sought. An indirect method of estimation is "a method to arrive at prevalence through the use of a documentary statistic known to vary with the rate of alcoholism" (16, p.294). Though other statistics have been used, the most common one has been the incidence of death due to cirrhosis of the liver. Cirrhosis is defined (17, p.320) as "a disease of the liver, marked by progressive destruction of liver cells, accompanied by regeneration of the liver substance and increase of connective tissue." One is left with a fibrotic, nodular, and (eventually) malfunctioning liver which is very characteristic in appearance upon either gross or microscopic examination and which in its advanced stages is incompatible with life. Cirrhosis may be due to several causes, but is most commonly seen in the end stages of chronic alcoholism.

There has been much discussion about the adequacy of cirrhosis deaths as an indicator of the prevalence of alcoholism. The original mathematical formula which expressed the relationship was developed by E. M. Jellinek, and has been subsequently modified. Popham and his co-workers (9, 16) feel that of all the indirect methods the original formula of Jellinek is the best. There have been 16 separate instances in which estimates derived from the Jellinek formula could be compared with independent methods of estimation. The results are impressively close (see especially 17, Table 39-2, p.300), with a linear correlation coefficient of .88, an extremely high value. Indeed, the correlation is so great that Popham has suggested the use of cirrhosis deaths directly instead of making the conversion when what one is interested in is spatial and temporal variation rather than absolute numbers. For absolute numbers he concludes the Jellinek formula is the best indirect indicator available (17, p.303). In summary, the correlation between the incidence of alcoholism and the incidence of death due to cirrhosis of the liver is extremely high.

This implies, but does not prove, that there would also be a high correlation between the per capita consumption of alcohol and the incidence of cirrhosis. Independent data are here available from a number of sources. Summarizing several of them, Popham (17, p.299) states that "all of the coefficients are statistically significant and are very large." Another Canadian observer (15) calculated a correlation of .96 between per capita consumption and cirrhosis for the adult population of his country between 1929 and 1956, a truly extraordinary finding.

More to the point for Pennsylvania is the exhaustive research carried out on a county-by-county basis by Dr. George K. Tokuhata and his associates of the division of research and biostatistics of the Pennsylvania Department of Health. They found (18) a direct correlation between alcohol consumption and death from cirrhosis which was as high as .87 in the lower socioeconomic counties of the state. They also found that persons dying of cirrhosis in Pennsylvania did so approximately 10 years before they would have been expected to die of other causes. The percentage risk of dying from cirrhosis was highest in the 25-29 year age group. Dr. Tokuhata and his colleagues were impressed with the possible relationship of nutrition to these findings. It had long been thought that malnutrition was necessary for the production of cirrhosis, as well as the excessive consumption of alcohol. Recent research in higher primates, as well as in human beings, indicates otherwise (19, 20); both pathological liver changes and deterioration of muscles were produced in the presence of a nutritionally adequate diet. Thus the relationship between the consumption of alcohol and the development of cirrhosis seems very well established, and may not require the additional presence of malnutrition.

Common sense would indicate that the correlation between the price of alcohol and the per capita consumption of alcohol would be high. But there is also research evidence that this is so. In his famous study of the relationship between the number of outlets for alcohol and alcohol consumption, Entine (21) noted that in areas where the median family income was high, package store sales tended to be high, whether or not there were a great many outlets or very few in relation to the population. The reverse was also true. Seeley (15) found a correlation of .99 between price and consumption.

In view of the high correlations between all of these factors it is reasonable to suppose that they are interconnected. The most striking evidence for this has been produced by the Canadians, who present graphic representations of the fact that, over the years, the price of alcohol relative to disposable income has gone steadily downhill, while both the per capita consumption of alcohol and the incidence of death due to cirrhosis have steadily climbed (9, 15). Although from a strictly technical point of view correlations do not prove causality, there is highly presumptive evidence here for a causal chain. In plain terms, when the price of alcohol goes down people buy more and drink more. As a result, more people become alcoholic and die of cirrhosis.

The evidence in favor of this proposition seems so strong that disagreement with it would appear unlikely. However, there are dissenting voices. This is very likely a function of the fact that the social sciences, unlike the physical sciences, are rarely exact. In most instances they can supply only approximate answers. The types of precise experiments which are possible with inert matter are rarely ethically feasible with living beings, particularly human beings. Therefore, proofs in the social sciences are rarely total and there is usually room for disagreement. This is why social science research can (and in our view must) contribute to the making of social policy but cannot determine social policy. In the absence of complete precision there is the need for the exercise of judgment; and in matters of human behavior, as complex as they are, that exercise of judgment is almost always called for.

Such is the case in the present instance. Mark Keller of Rutgers basically disagrees with the price mechanism hypothesis. In view of his eminence in the field and his position as editor of the *Quarterly Journal of Studies in Alcohol,* his dissent must be heard. Accordingly, it is reproduced in full in the appended materials (see Appendix C). We are grateful to Mr. Keller for having taken the time to respond so fully to our requests for his opinion.

Basically, the disagreement between Keller and the Canadians amounts to a disagreement as to the nature of alcoholism. Keller believes that the "proto-alcoholic" discovers in alcohol "a practically magical pharmacological effect" and does not believe that many "will fail to discover their magic pharmacon just because the government has made it more inconvenient to get the stuff. Not so long as they can get it at all." This notion is based on the disease concept of alcohol, something which Keller readily espouses (p.3). He concludes, with respect to the price mechanism, that "it wouldn't work at all in the U.S.A., certainly not in the latter part of the twentieth century" (p.2).

Keller believes that the Canadian researchers would agree with him about the disease nature of alcohol. In fact they do not (9, pp. 12-15 - see Appendix B).* They stigmatize his view as one which derives directly from the Temperance Movement. There has been of late a good deal of criticism of the disease concept from other quarters as well. For example, the Addiction Research Unit at the Maudsley Hospital in London under Dr. Griffith Edwards not long ago contributed an elegant article to Mr. Keller's own journal on precisely this issue (22). In the opinion of this reviewer, the weight of the empirical evidence is strongly on the side of the Canadians and against the disease concept of

* Mr. Popham's instructions were that his paper could be distributed only on a limited basis. Since Mr. Keller is a journal editor, it did not seem reasonable to distribute the paper to him. As the paper has not yet been published, Mr. Keller has not seen it. Hence he is unaware of the disagreement.

alcoholism. Keller's view is surprisingly out of date and reinforced with almost no hard data. But much of the material upon which these differing views are based is to be found in the appendices, and readers are urged to read it and consider for themselves.

Implications of the Price Mechanism

If the Canadian researchers are correct, or are as nearly correct as one can be in the social science field, then it follows that, short of heroic and probably unworkable alternatives such as total or near-total prohibition, the only effective mechanism which government policy can employ to diminish alcoholism is the price mechanism. That is the government must raise the price of alcohol to the point where sales and consumption drop. If the government fails to do this, it is highly probable that the incidence of alcoholism will continue to rise as the price of alcohol continues to fall.

It may be argued in rebuttal that the government badly requires the sort of revenue which would result from increased sales of alcohol, whether under public or private auspices. Much evidence suggests, however, that this would be a short-sighted (if temporarily effective) way to obtain funds. In the end the government will pay out in the costs of dealing with problems of alcoholism as much or more than it realizes on the increased sales. For the costs of alcoholism are horrendous. In terms of police time alone, the Moreland Commission estimated that at least 60% of all arrests are directly related to problems of alcoholism (3, p.23). Not only does this represent a considerable public cost, but to it must be added the cost of the crime which is committed because of the diversion of police attention. There are many other costs, such as those involved in hospital care of alcoholics, in traffic accidents caused by alcoholics, and so forth. Society will pay, one way or another.

This viewpoint has been eloquently summarized by H. David Archibald, vice-chairman of the Addiction Research Foundation of Ontario. Among the points made by Mr. Archibald to emphasize the costs of alcohol were the following (this material is a paraphrase and not necessarily a direct quotation):

> *France has the highest consumption of alcohol in the world. The average Frenchman drinks 25 liters of absolute alcohol a year, compared to about nine liters for the average adult in Ontario. While some people praise the integration of alcohol into the daily life of the French and would like to emulate this "continental" pattern of drinking, there are serious drawbacks. France also has the world's highest death rate from cirrhosis of the liver, about six times that in Canada. Forty-two percent of the total health expenditures in France are attributable to the treatment of alcohol-*

> *related disease, and about 50% of all hospital beds are occupied by such patients.*
>
> *In Ontario, alcohol related problems are responsible for more than 10% of expenditures in the general public hospitals, more than 15% in mental hospitals, approximately 20% of the expenditures under the Family Benefits Act, and 30% of expenditures for Children's Aid Societies. This means that the Ontario taxpayer (in 1971) paid $89 million through the Ontario Hospital Insurance Plan for illness relating to alcoholism; he paid almost $17 million through the mental hospital system; almost $9 million through the Family Benefits Act, and over $11 million through the Children's Aid Societies for activities attributable to alcoholism.*
>
> *The taxpayer paid more than $134 million in one year for illness and disruption attributed directly to alcoholism. This figure does* not *include physician's fees, municipal welfare payments, the enormous cost to business and industry through loss of productivity and manpower; nor does it reflect the fact that alcohol is involved in over 50% of deaths due to traffic accidents in Canada (23, pp. 7-8, 10).*

Implementation of a policy of control of alcoholism by exercise of the price mechanism in the Commonwealth of Pennsylvania would certainly present serious problems. Not the least of these would be the ready availability of alcohol beverages in jurisdictions immediately accessible to Pennsylvanians. Even as this report is being written, stories appear in the newspaper headlined "Higher Prices Spiriting Away Liquor Sales" (Philadelphia *Inquirer,* Sunday, December 2, 1973, p. 12-B). They claim that as much as $25 million in lost tax revenues are flowing from Pennsylvania pockets into the treasuries of neighboring states because of the relatively high liquor prices in the Commonwealth. It may be easy to police the borders of the Province of Ontario, which are either sparsely populated or of international character, or the borders of a country like Finland, which artifically inflates its retail alcohol prices. But it is *not* easy to police the traffic coming over the Ben Franklin and Walt Whitman bridges into Philadelphia.

Moreover, there is the problem of the state monopoly itself. There must be something wrong with it. Whereas in aggregate state store prices are lower in monopoly states than in license states (4, 12, 13) this does not seem to be the case in Pennsylvania. A feeling has grown that perhaps the simplest thing would be for the state to get out of the liquor business and place retail sales back into private hands. It is interesting that this is not the first time such an issue has been raised. In 1934 George H. Earle succeeded Governor Pinchot, who had established the state monopoly. He was the first Democratic governor of Pennsylvania in 35 years. No sooner had he taken office than he stated publicly that liquor prices in Pennsylvania were "absolutely outrageous compared with prices paid in other states." He called for an investigation. A special committee was formed and eventually recommended not only a continuance of the monopoly but a tightening of its controls (4, pp. 15-16).

Unfortunately, there is every indication that disposal of the state stores would materially increase the problems of alcoholism in Pennsylvania. There would be a direct effect through the price mechanism. Retail prices would immediately be lowered, both as a result of outlets competing with those in other states and competing with each other in Pennsylvania. With the lowered price, consumption of alcohol and therefore alcoholism would inevitably increase.

But the long-term results would be even more unfortunate. Disposal of the state stores to private licensees would at a stroke create a powerful vested interest in maintaining the price of alcohol at the lowest possible level, not only at the present time but in perpetuity. This is probably the principle reason for not disposing of the state store system. The fear of a vested interest is not a recent fear. As long ago as 1934 Smith (5) noted an immediate clamor when New Hampshire created its State Store system: "...the druggists, restaurant owners, small hotel owners, and advertisers want the law and its administration liberalized in the direction of their particular interests." The anonymous author of "Medicolegal Notes" in 1940 was more direct: "...the inevitable result of the license system has been the entrance of liquor interests into politics through legislative lobbies to secure relaxation of restrictions and protect their interests as business enterprises" (6, p.565). Twiley Barker noted that "the loudest complaints come from groups primarily composed of those who would be in the liquor business if it were not operated by the state ... there has been no evidence of widespread public dissatisfaction, and no state which has adopted the plan in the post-Prohibition period has subsequently abandoned it" (2, p.501).

There is every reason to fear that the vested interest created would be both vocal and politically influential. It would have the active backing of the national alcoholic beverage industry. Thus disposal of the state stores would deprive the government of the Commonwealth permanently of what may be the only effective policy measure it can take against the ever-increasing tide of alcoholism: the manipulation of the price mechanism. Responsible governmental officials must weigh the loss of the price mechanism against the difficulties which would ensue in using it. There may be other factors which this report has not considered, political factors among them. But according to our current understanding the weight of the evidence favors retention of the state stores and the use of the price mechanism to control the problem of alcoholism.

Some Mitigating Factors

There are steps which might be taken to make implementing the price mechanism less problematic. First and foremost is the education of the public. One is entitled to wonder whether an informed public would continue to view alcohol as just another commodity which they must obtain at the lowest possible price. One is entitled to wonder whether a public appraised of the very real and very severe dangers of alcohol consumption would go charging over the Jersey bridges and down the coast to Plain Old Pearson's to cart back bottles of booze.

A major part of such a public information campaign should include the education of the public as to the total costs to society of alcoholism, and the likelihood that those costs will increase if measures are not taken against alcoholism. This aspect of the educational process should most properly be based upon a careful audit of these expenses, so that data similar to that cited by Archibald could be made available for Pennsylvania and at today's inflated prices. If it were shown that, in Pennsylvania as well as in Ontario, whatever increased revenue the public might realize by making alcohol more available would be lost, perhaps several times over, by the resultant costs, and if the public was aware of the fact that it was losing money on the deal, one is entitled to doubt it would opt for the greater availability of alcohol.

The evolution of the thinking of the individual preparing this report may be instructive. He was disposed hitherto to view the state liquor monopoly as an example of moral leprosy that all right-thinking statesmen would eradicate at the earliest opportunity. It was wrong, he felt, for the state of profit from the miseries of others. But since it now appears on more careful consideration that the state monopoly system could be employed to good effect, he has changed his mind. Others might do likewise. In sum, a well-constructed public education campaign which would result in Pennsylvanians viewing alcohol as a major public health hazard might well offset many of the supposed disadvantages of the use of the price mechanism. The establishment of a single state agency, which could superintend such a campaign, has already been an important contribution of the current administration.

There is another, more practical possibility which should be seriously considered. The Canadian researchers point out that it is unlikely the public would sit still for an increment in the price of alcohol which would flow into the general fund. This is especially true in contemporary America, where scandals at the federal level have made skeptics of the most trusting souls. No doubt such a move would be seen as being insincere and as motivated only by the government's desire for more revenues, to be used for such things as enhancing the salaries and perquisites of state officials. The public already is desperately conscious of the tax bite and tends to feel that government gets enough. Several states have already adopted a mechanism which could answer this doubt by demonstrating that, rather than raising funds for other and unspecified purposes, the government was serious about its war on alcoholism.

This mechanism consists in dedicating the funds raised by the increased tax to the treatment and prevention of alcoholism. The logic of this position seems unassailable. It has long been established that the ingestion of alcohol is a privilege, not a right. This is implicit in the existence of controls over alcohol and is entirely justified by its harmfulness. The tax would bring home, as no other method could, the obligations which are incurred by citizens who exercise the privilege of consuming alcohol. The government agrees to make the substance available to them, but only under the condition that they recognize that some individuals, not necessarily themselves, are being harmed by its availability, and that they have obligation to provide both for the treatment of these individuals and for educational and other preventive methods which will keep the vulnerable person from harm.

Coincidentally the tax would, of course, raise the price of alcohol and exert a preventive effect thereby. As nearly as could be determined within the time constraints of this study, 12 states have taken this route or one similar to it. Four options generally are used, each state exercising a single option with the exception of the state of Washington, which exercises two. The options include financing alcoholism treatment, prevention, education, and rehabilitation from (1) a special tax; (2) license fees paid for the sale of alcohol; (3) a percentage of the profits realized on the retail sale of alcohol; or (4) an appropriation derived from the overall alcohol revenues realized by the state from all sources. The first option is exercised by Michigan, North Carolina, South Carolina, and South Dakota; the second by the District of Columbia, Indiana, Ohio, and the state of Washington; the third by Virginia and the state of Washington; and the fourth by Alabama, Vermont, and Wisconsin. These data are presented in tabular form in Table 1, Appendix D.

Of all of these taxes, the most interesting appears to be that of South Carolina. This state previously did not permit the on-premises sale of alcohol. It also maintained a monopoly over package sales. In 1973, a constitutional amendment was passed which permitted the sale of alcohol for on-premises consumption with fairly strict regulations, including the provision that the alcohol could be sold only in sealed containers of two ounces or less. For this reason it is commonly referred to as the "minibottle legislation." The constitutional amendment was passed in conjunction with another law, which stipulates as follows:

> *Twenty-five percent of revenue derived under the provisions of this act shall be returned to the countries on a per capita basis according to the latest official United States census, to be used for educational purposes relating to the use of alcoholic liquors and for the rehabilitation of alcoholics*

and drug addicts. Counties may pool such funds with other counties and with other funds for these purposes. (Section 5 of Act 1063 of 1973).

Copies of the relevant South Carolina enactments and of our correspondence with the South Carolina Commission on Alcoholism are appended to this report (Appendix E). Because of the recency of the legislation it is not possible to gauge its effects as yet. South Carolina has kindly agreed to keep us informed on a continuing basis of its experience. We have also requested similar information and copies of legislation from all other states engaged in this form of taxation. As yet this material has not arrived; it will be forwarded when it does.

We feel that the dedicated tax mechanism is an extremely appealing one from many points of view. Further study of the experience in South Carolina and elsewhere will be helpful in determining whether its application to Pennsylvania is justified. There appears to be no compelling reason why it should not be. We have been warned by one of our contacts that the liquor industry does not look kindly upon such earmarking of funds and would probably lobby against it and defeat it as it did in Maryland. (Our information from Maryland is rather different, and indicates it is probable that the legislature there will soon pass such a law.) This same source indicates that, notwithstanding this view, the liquor industry finds some kinds of earmarking more acceptable than others. An offer was made to contact the highest councils of the industry on a trial basis to gauge their reaction to whatever Pennsylvania may be considering. We feel that this offer should be viewed with some reservations.

Implementation of any or all of these plans would be far more readily done if other states in the mid-Atlantic region could be involved in a concerted and uniform attempt than if Pennsylvania acted alone. This administration has previously suggested such cooperation with respect to dealing with the problem of narcotics. If there seems to be some community of feeling based on this prior experience, perhaps Pennsylvania could take the lead in a sound regional approach to this problem.

In conclusion, we recognize that retention of the state liquor monopoly and the use of a categorical tax to raise the price of alcoholism as a public health measure is not likely to be a popular policy, or one that is easy to follow. We further recognize that many other factors of which we are not aware may enter into the deliberations on this matter and be decisive in one way or another. Nevertheless, we are satisfied that on the basis of the evidence known to us it is the most prudent policy to follow in the long run. We look forward to discussing these materials with interested officials of the state government, and hope that the input of this report may be helpful to them in their difficult task.

References

1. Raffalovich, Alexis. The state monopoly of spirits in Russia, and its influence on the prosperity of the population. *J. Royal Statistical Soc., 64:* 1-30 (Mar.), 1901.

2. Barker, Twiley W., Jr. The states in the liquor business: Some observations on administration. *Quart. J. Stud. Alcohol, 18:* 492-502, 1957.

3. Bacon, Selden D., and Jones, R.W. The relationship of the alcoholic beverage control law and the problem of alcohol. Study Paper No. 1 of the New York State Moreland Commission on the Alcoholic Beverage Control Law. Second Edition (revised). October 18th, 1963.

4. McGeary, M. Nelson. *Pennsylvania and the Liquor Business.* State College, Pennsylvania, Penns Valley Publishers, 1948.

5. Smith, Milton V. Early administrative phases of a state liquor store system. *American Political Sci. Rev., 28:* 1064-71, 1934.

6. Anonymous. Medicolegal notes: State control of trade in alcoholic beverages. *Quart. J. Stud. Aclohol, 1:* 563-81 (Dec.), 1940.

7. Landis, Benson Y. Economic aspects of state alcoholic beverage monopoly enterprises, 1937-1946. *Quart. J. Stud. Alcohol, 9:* 259-69, 1948.

8. Orlans, Harold. Making social research more useful to government. *Social Science Information, 7:* 151-58, 1968.

9. Popham, Robert E., Schmidt, Wolfgang, and deLint, Jan. The prevention of alcoholism: Epidemiological studies of the effects of government control measures. Manuscript. To be published in: Ewing, J.A., and Rouse, B.A. (Eds.): *Law and Drinking Behavior,* Chapel Hill, University of North Carolina Press. Ms. received 9/7/73.

10. Anonymous. Federal taxation of state liquor monopolies. Harvard Law Review, 47: 32—25, 1933.

11. Keller, Mark. A review of Denny, Edgar M. *State Liquor Control: Monopoly and License Systems.* Institute of Government, University of Utah, Bull. Ser. No. 8, Salt Lake City, March 1950. *Quart. J. Stud. Alcohol, 14:* 122-23 (March), 1953.

12. Lohrke, G. A comparison of operations between selected municipal and private liquor dispensaries in Minnesota. Ph.D. dissertation, University of Oklahoma, 1968. (University Microfilms No. 68-14, 205.) Source of abstract: *Diss. Abstr.* 29:B-1012, 1968. Reviewed in *Quart. J. Stud. Alcohol, 30:* 808-09 (Sept.), 1969.

13. Simon, Julian L. The economic effects of state monopoly on packaged-liquor retailing. *J. Political Economy, 74:* 188-94, 1966.

14. Jellinek, E.M. Recent trends in alcoholism and in alcohol consumption. *Quart. J. Stud. Alcohol, 8:* 1-42, 1947.

15. Seeley, John R. Death by liver cirrhosis and the price of beverage alcohol. *Canad. Med. Assn. J., 83:* 1361-66, (Dec. 24) 1960.

16. Popham, Robert E. Indirect methods of alcoholism prevalence estimation: A critical evaluation. *In: Alcohol and Alcoholism,* ed. Robert E. Popham, Toronto, University of Toronto Press, 1970, pp. 294-306.

17. Dorland, W.A. Newman. *The American Illustrated Medical Dictionary,* 22nd Edition. Philadelphia, W.B. Saunders Company, 1951.

18. Tokuhata, George K., Digon, Edward, and Ramaswamy, Krishna. Alcohol sales and socioeconomic factors related to cirrhosis of the liver mortality in Pennsylvania. *HSMHA Health Reports, 86:* 253-64 (March) 1971.

19. Rubin, Emanuel, and Lieber, Charles S. Experimental alcoholic hepatitis: A new primate model. *Science, 182:* 712-13 (Nov.16) 1973.

20. Song, Sun K., and Rubin, Emanuel. Ethanol produces muscle damage in human volunteers. *Science, 175:* 327-28 (Jan. 21) 1972.

21. Entine, Alan D. The relationship between the number of sales outlets and the consumption of alcoholic beverages in New York and other states. Study Paper No. 2 of the New York State Moreland Commission on the Alcoholic Beverage Control Law. Second Edition. October 21, 1963.

22. Robinson, David. The alcohologist's addiction: Some implications of having lost control over the disease concept of alcoholism. *Quart. J. Stud. Alcohol, 33:* 1028-59 (Dec.) 1972.

23. Archibald, H. David. Changing drinking patterns in Ontario—some implications. *Addictions, 20* (3):2-17, (Fall) 1973.

ERRATA

Foreword

p. ix	para. 3	l. 2	"the" primary
p. xii	footnote	l. 1	"Freda" Adler

Introduction

p. xix	para. 1	l. 16	"the" major

Chapter 1

p. 4	para. 1	l. 1	encounters "with alcohol"
p. 5		l. 6	"'till" 'tis
p. 5	para. 2	l. 16	"Sertürner"
p. 19	table		Annual Absolute Alcohol Equivalents
		col. 3	Pennsylvania
		col. 4	Assumed Absolute Alcohol Content**
p. 25	para. 2	l. 10	Chapter "13"

Chapter 3

p. 51	para. 1	l. 4	passage "in"

Chapter 4

p. 61	para. 2	l. 5	"were" not gathered

Chapter 5

p. 76	para. 1	l. 8	"treatment"
p. 80	para. 1	l. 33	In "contrast"
p. 81	para. 1	l. 14	"excessive"
p. 88		col. 4	"county"
p. 100	para. 3	l. 5	"county"

Chapter 6

p. 111	para. 2	l. 33	"their" function
p. 114		l. 6	"in" out-patient

Chapter 7

References:

1. Osmond, H. Function as the basis of psychiatric ward design. In: Proshansky, Harold M., William H. Ittelson, and Leanne G. Rivlin (eds.): Environmental Psychology: Man and His Physical Setting. New York, Holt, Rinehart & Winston, 1970, pp. 560-69.

2. Root, Laura E. Social therapies in the treatment of alcoholics. In: Pittman, David J. (ed.): Alcoholism. New York, Harper & Row, 1967, pp. 142-56.

3. Ittelson, William H., Harold M. Proshansky, and Leanne G. Rivlin, The environmental psychology of the psychiatric ward. In: Proshansky, Harold M., William H. Ittelson, and Leanne G. Rivlin (eds.): Environmental Psychology: Man and His Physical Setting. New York, Holt, Rinehart & Winston, 1970, pp. 419-39.

4. Root, Laura E. op. cit.

5. Adler, F., Moffett, A.D., Glaser, F.B., et al. A Systems Approach to Drug Treatment. Philadelphia, Dorrance & Company, 1974.

Chapter 8

p. 125	para. 2	l. 10	"were" thought

Chapter 9

p. 128	para. 2	l. 3	"treatment"
p. 132	para. 1	l. 2	"qua"
p. 132	para. 2	l. 11	"other"
p. 134	para. 1	l. 6	may not be "overwhelmingly popular"

Chapter 10

p. 138	para. 2	l. 4	"consensus"

Chapter 11

p. 147	para. 1	l. 9	delete "substantial"
p. 147	para. 4	l. 9	patient "increases"

Chapter 13

p. 165	para. 1	l. 6	"Ebby" T.
p. 166		l. 3	"Ebby" T.
p. 169	para. 1	l. 18	delete second ","
p. 173	para. 2	l. 4	"demographic" survey

Chapter 14

p. 187	para. 3	l. 5,6	"was a" college "graduate"

Chapter 15

p. 191		l. 14	"affective"

Acknowledgements

p. 280	para. 1	l. 10	"Greenberg"

Government Policy and the Problem of Alcoholism

p. 284	para. 1	l. 11	"causal"
p. 291		l. 5	"vehicle"